THE PREVENTION
of
CROHN'S DISEASE

Gilles R. G. Monif M.D.

authorHOUSE®

AuthorHouse™
1663 Liberty Drive
Bloomington, IN 47403
www.authorhouse.com
Phone: 1 (800) 839-8640

Published by AuthorHouse   09/10/2015

ISBN: 978-1-5049-2310-1 (sc)
ISBN: 978-1-5049-2309-5 (e)

Library of Congress Control Number: 2015911199

Print information available on the last page.

DEDICATION

To Karel Hruska and Ivo Pavlik who spoke out when others sinned by silence.

PREFACE

Citizens have enduring moral right to the resources that govern their survival. Within the public trust, they have the moral and legal authority to demand that their rights be upheld.

The concept of the public trust is not a nebulous idealistic concept. The public trust is an area of law for which government is its trustee. Deliberately withholding information that an adulterated product may be hazardous to the public health transgresses the fine line between civil and criminal negligence.

Crohn's disease is more than a destroyer of life. Directly or indirectly, Crohn's disease kills.

Table of Contents

Part I

CROHN'S DISEASE

Part II

SINNING BY SILENCE

APPENDIX

Part I

CROHN'S DISEASE

WHAT IS CROHN'S DISEASE?

- **Crohn's disease is an inflammatory disease of the human gastrointestinal tract.** The primary regions affected are the small bowel and the first portion of the large bowel.

- The disease causes affected individuals to precipitously seek a bathroom many times a day.

- One in four afflicted individuals will have one or more surgeries to remove diseased bowel.

- **The characteristic time of onset is between 11-24 years of age.** A second, smaller disease group occurs at a time of waning immunity late in life.

- **The early onset of Crohn's disease progressively tends to involve more children**.

- For most afflicted individuals, Crohn's disease is a life-long affliction.

- In 2002, the Centers for Disease Control and Prevention (CDC) had placed the number of US cases of Crohn's disease at 200,000. **By 2010, there were over 800,000 cases of Crohn's disease in**

the United States and over 1.5 million cases in westernized countries.

- Certain ethnic populations appear to have a greater predisposition to the disease than other ethnic groups.

- As the economies of third world countries have improved, the prevalence of Crohn's disease in these populations has dramatically increased.

- **In the United States, the medical costs to an individual afflicted with Crohn's disease are $12,000-$18,000 a year.**

- The United States' annual medical and indirect costs from Crohn's disease are estimated to be over **$10 billion** and **$4.2 billion respectively.**

- Crohn's disease causes a significant number of afflicted individuals, in the midst of their most important earning years, to prematurely leave the work force or change employment to accommodate the demands of the disease. The progressively increasing medical costs of Crohn's disease are being assumed by the federal government.

- The number of new cases of Crohn's disease per year is increasing worldwide. **The burning question is "Why?"**

ZOONOTIC BRIDGES

Dorland's Medical Dictionary defines zoonosis (zoo plus the Greek *nosos* meaning disease) as a disease of animals that may be transmitted to man under natural conditions. The term, zoonotic, means an infection of an animal being transmittable to humans.

Historically, the United States Department of Agriculture (USDA) has given special attention to micro-organisms that have negative effects on agriculture and agriculture-dependent businesses. When agriculture-based, zoonotic pathogens threaten a significant element within agribusiness, USDA has been prompt to act to destroy the transmission bridge between the source and man.

Two prime examples of USDA's interventions when the public health had been threatened have been brucellosis and bovine tuberculosis due to *Brucella abortus and Mycobacterium bovis*, respectively.

The brucella organism was transmitted to humans through wool and animal contact. USDA instituted a policy (test-and-cull) in which each animal within the herd was tested and those that tested positive for brucella antigens were removed from the herd and destroyed.

Cows infected with *M. bovis* had the potential to shed viable organisms into unpasteurized milk. When ingested in sufficient quantity, this mycobacterium produces chronic enteritis that is not dissimilar to that characteristic of Crohn's disease. The threat to agriculture was deemed so significant that when an animal was documented to be infected, not only was it destroyed, but so were all of its herd mates.

MILK

Milk is critical in conveying nutrition and immunity from a female to its offspring. In nutritionally stressed countries, survival of an infant is largely influenced by the age the child is weaned in order to feed the next baby.

Perception of the nutritional value of milk has resulted in the rearing of animals (cows, goats, sheep, camels etc.) for the express purpose of providing a food source for human consumption.

In 1863, Louis Pasteur found that if he heated the local grapes to about 50-80 degrees Centigrade for a brief period of time, he could prevent the wine from souring. The occasional presence of pathogenic microbes in milk fostered the adoption of pasteurization.

Pasteurization does not kill all the microbes present in milk. What it does is reduce the number of organisms, thereby allowing the taste of the milk not to be impaired until after a calculated expiration date. High-temperature, short-time (HTST) pasteurized milk typically has a refrigerated shelf life of two-three weeks. HTST pasteurization is designed to achieve a five-log reduction, killing 99.999% of bacteria such as salmonella, listeria, campylobacter, *Staphylococcus aureus,* pathogenic *Escherichia coli* and *Mycobacterium bovis* among others. Ultra-pasteurized milk can last longer.

Gilles R. G. Monif M.D.

The set point for temperature and duration of pasteurization is determined by the pathogenic micro-organism that can potentially contaminate or be shed into milk.

One of the most important milk-related pathogen had been *Mycobacterium bovis*.

MYOCOBACTERIUM BOVIS

Mycobacterium. bovis is the main cause of tuberculosis in cattle and other mammals. Infection/disease is acquired by oral ingestion of the organism resulting in gastrointestinal disease as its primary clinical manifestation.

The eighteenth century fashion of very high collars covering the entire neck resulted from non-tuberculous, mycobacterial infection of the neck lymph nodes causing disfiguring masses and fistulae (scrofula).

U.S. figures for deaths (pre-pasteurization) due to *M. bovis* have been difficult to obtain. Between 1912 and 1937, an estimated 65,000 individuals in England and Wales died from the disease of the gastrointestinal tract contracted from the consumption of milk containing *M. bovis*.

This threat to the public welfare was ultimately resolved when it was demonstrated that *M. bovis* could be destroyed by proper pasteurization.

Gilles R. G. Monif M.D.

MYCOBACTERIUM AVIUM SUBSPECIES PARATUBERCULOSIS

Modern day mycobacterium groupings are the result of their divergence through an apparent evolutionary bottleneck. *Mycobacterium avium* subspecies *paratuberculosis* is presumed to be derived from *Mycobacterium avium* or possibly *Mycobacterium hominissuis.* Being a relatively newer strain, MAP exhibits greater disease producing potential than *M. avium.*

MAP has a near global presence in soil. MAP can become embedded in the food supply of animals that eat grass and plants. MAP infection has been identified in almost every herbivore studied in depth: cows, sheep, goats, deer, elk, buffalo, camels etc. Animals such as rabbits that share pasture with infected animals can become infected and disseminate the organism beyond the confines of a given pasture.

Animals become infected by consuming plant material or water containing MAP. In animals whose immune systems are not able to inhibit continued MAP reproduction, infection progresses to a chronic granulomatous infection of their gastrointestinal tract. In cattle, the resultant disease is called **paratuberculosis** or **Johne's disease**. Animals with progressive infection develop soft stools that eventually progress to profuse diarrhea. Animals with active infection produce less milk, have poorer reproductive outcomes, and lower slaughter weight. If allowed to run its course, Johne's disease is usually terminal. On a global level, MAP infection/disease of domesticated milk producing animals is a multi-billion dollar problem for producers.

Like *Mycobacterium tuberculosis*, in rare cases, MAP crosses the placental barrier, causing infection of the baby while it is in its mother's womb.

Once MAP is introduced into the pasture environment, elimination of the organism is extraordinarily difficult. Even if elimination of MAP could be achieved, the ultimate reservoirs of infection cannot be easily eradicated. Within a confined herd, once a resident animal develops clinical signs, a significant number of animals within the herd will have already been infected.

The gastrointestinal tract of animals, as well as humans, contains complementary receptor sites that allow MAP to attach to the mucosa. The universal presence of these receptor sites has explained the ease with which MAP can cross species barriers. The MAP of a goat or an elk can infect cows and humans and vice versa. **Human MAP isolates have similar genetic markers to animal MAP isolates.**

The primary concern of USDA and veterinary medicine has been reducing the economic cost to producers from MAP induced diseases.

CROHN'S DISEASE

Crohn's disease is a chronic granulomatous inflammation of the human gastrointestinal tract. The primary areas affected are the small and the proximal portion of the large bowel.

Individuals with Crohn's disease experience the sudden, often explosive, need to defecate many times a day. The development of bowel obstruction, bowel perforation, fistula formation or abscess formation will require one in four afflicted individuals to have one or more surgeries to remove diseased bowel.

For most individuals, Crohn's disease is a lifelong affliction. It causes a significant number of afflicted individuals in the midst of their most productive earning years to prematurely leave the work force or change their employment to accommodate the demands of the disease.

The United States is in the midst of a Crohn's disease epidemic. According to the National Association for Colitis and Crohn's disease, in 2001, Crohn's disease affected about one in every 1,600 individuals. In 2002, the CDC estimated the number of afflicted individuals to be 200,000.

By 2010, the number of cases of Crohn's disease in the United States was estimated to be 800,000. A more recent estimate places the number of cases above one million.

If the number of U.S. cases cited by sources in the United Kingdom is accurate, a more realistic figure may be 1.2

million. Along with the increased number of cases, the onset of disease has shifted towards an earlier age.

The United States is not alone in experiencing an epidemic. An additional 1.5 - 2.0 million cases of Crohn's disease exist in other westernized countries. As the economies of third world countries have shifted to western style diet, the incidence of Crohn's disease has substantially increased.

In the United States, the annual medical cost is conservatively estimated to be over $10 billion. No indirect/societal costs of Crohn's disease have been published to date. The burden of payment is increasingly shifting to the federal government.

HYPOTHESIS

A hypothesis is an upscale word for a well thought out guess. In medicine, most sophisticated guesses/hypotheses are derived from observations derived from experiments in nature.

Being pure sciences, the laws within mathematics or physics always render the same answer. Medicine is not a pure science.

Medicine is a pseudo-science. Its facts are never identical. The foundations of its so-called "scientific truths" are, more often than not, the residues of coinciding probabilities. Much of medicine is conjectural science, based upon statistics which serve as empirical enumeration of observations.

The French physiologist, Claude Bernard, wrote *"the application of mathematics to natural phenomena is the aim of all science"*. He went on to state that attempts to apply mathematics to medical problems were flawed because the empirical data would always be insufficient. He therefore held that instead of trying to reduce to equations the facts that are already known, the most useful pathway for medicine to follow was to seek to discover new facts.

In his classical work, ***The Study of Experimental Medicine,*** Professor Bernard describes the guidelines by which conjecture becomes a "scientific truth".

To translate an observation in nature to a pseudo-scientific fact, involves four steps:

- Gather all the information relevant to the observation under analysis.

- Construct a hypothesis to account for the proposed postulate relating to the observation.

- Construct an experimental design to, not support the hypothesis, but **challenge** the hypothesis.

- Reinterpret the hypothesis in light of the data.

An unwritten part of Claude Bernard's scientific method is that the exceptions must prove the prevailing "scientific truth".

****

The hypothesis of causality linking MAP and Crohn's disease was advanced by John Hermon-Taylor. He described a case of a young boy with scrofula from which MAP was recovered. Subsequently, the boy went on to develop Crohn's disease. Seizing upon this observation, Hermon-Taylor and his collaborators have gone on and produced an impressive body of work in support of this hypothesis.

Working within the veterinary sciences, Ron Chiodini noted the similarity in the histopathology of Johne's disease due to *Mycobacterium avium* subspecies *paratuberculosis* (MAP) in herbivores and the histopathology of Crohn's disease in humans. In 1989, Chiodini published a review and comparison of Crohn's disease in humans and of Johne's disease in cattle.

A major difference between the histopathology of Johne's disease in cattle and Crohn's disease in humans is that, while MAP DNA can be demonstrated in diseased human tissues, special stains do not demonstrate the presence of acid-fast bacilli; nor does the organism grow out on solid media. This disconnect between the presence of MAP DNA, culture recovery, and histological demonstration of a mycobacterium was partially addressed by the demonstration that when isolated, MAP persisted as a spheroclast. The absence of a stainable outer coat prevented MAP's identification by special stains. Culture recovery required media that supports recovery of the spheroclastic form of MAP. Such media differs significantly from the solid agar used to isolate MAP from animals with Johne's disease. These differences between the two disease entities were significant.

In 1996, Chiodini and Rossiter isolated MAP from the feces of 26 out of 135 patients with Crohn's disease, but from only one of 121 control individuals. Previously, MAP had been assumed to be but an opportunistic human pathogen causing disease in, primarily but not exclusively, individuals whose immune system had been significantly impaired by a retrovirus (AIDS).

Chiodini and Rossiter's experimental design was to compare the presence of MAP in the stool of individuals with and without Crohn's disease. While circumstantially supporting the hypothesis of causality, the results were far from being incriminating. Guilt by association is not proof. Changes induced by a disease process can significantly alter the gastrointestinal tract's microbiological flora. It was argued that the tissue destruction observed in Crohn's disease had selected for the retention of MAP.

A "scientific truth" must address its exceptions. The 1996 isolation of MAP from a non-diseased individual was the exception that would eventually demand an answer.

The embers of the MAP/Crohn's disease controversy simmered until scientific publications documented the presence of viable MAP organisms in **pasteurized milk**. Demonstration of a pathogenic mycobacterium in milk opened Pandora's Box.

When any issue concerning food safety is identified, the societal response is spelled out by the **Rio Declaration on Food Safety and the Sanitary** and **Phytosanitary Measures of the World Trade Organization**.

The Rio Declaration on Food Safety. Principle 15 of the Rio Declaration states: *"In order to protect the environment, the precautionary approach shall be widely applied by States according to their capabilities. Where there are threats of serious or irreversible damage, lack of full knowledge shall not be used as a reason for postponing cost-effective measures to prevent environmental degradation"*.

The World Trade Organization Agreement on Sanitary and Phytosanitary Measures. Article 5.7 allows regulatory measures *"where relevant scientific evidence is insufficient to demonstrate the safety of a product or commodity"*.

In 1997, a group of USDA scientists headed by Judith Stabel published a paper claiming that the high temperature, short duration method of pasteurization used in the United States destroyed MAP. Irene Grant, among others, strongly criticized the methodology. The USDA scientists had taken frozen MAP organisms and then sonicated them prior to adulterating milk samples with the organisms. By so doing, they thereby created a predictable outcome. Despite significant scientific criticism, USDA never issued a retraction of its findings. When congressional hearings were held to determine if MAP constituted a public health hazard. The Food and Drug Administration (FDA) used this paper to reassure Congress that pasteurized milk in the United States was safe.

Subsequently, when milk was taken from regional grocery stores in the five most important dairy states, using relatively insensitive isolation technology, over 2% of the containers were documented to have cultivable MAP.

In May of 1999, the National Institute of Allergy and Infectious Diseases (NIAID) published its research agenda in which it targeted seeking an infectious cause of Crohn's disease as a possible research objective. This topic went unfunded by Congress.

In 2000, Naser and co-workers isolated MAP from the milk of two lactating women with Crohn's disease and none from samples from five normal control women. The number of critical observations would have been ridiculously small where it not for the source from which MAP was recovered.

MAP in feces is of limited significance. MAP in breast milk says systemic invasion.

Responding to this added piece of information, the CDC is said to have unsuccessfully explored the possibility of obtaining funding in order to identify risk factors for human disease.

Gilles R. G. Monif M.D.

RESPONSE TO A HYPOTHETICAL RISK

Lord Justice Phillips' 2001 report to Her Majesty's Government states *"Where the likelihood of a risk to human life may appear remote, where there is uncertainty, all reasonably practical precautions should be taken ...... **The importance of precautionary measures should not be played down on the grounds that the risk is unproven"**.*

By 2001, the Office International des Epizooties (OIE) had already listed paratuberculosis as a category B pathogen in terms of its socioeconomic and/or public health importance.

In June 2001, the United Kingdom Food Standard Agency issued its report for food standards. The conclusion statement contained the following language *"**There is undoubtedly sufficient cause for concern** (relative to MAP as being the cause of Crohn's disease) **for further action to be taken urgently to determine what the available data means** ...... This question can be divided into two areas: What action should be taken to reduce exposure to MAP even though the causal link is not established; and what action can be taken to increase the knowledge base so that future decisions may be based upon more information".*

In 2000-2001, the United States Congress held hearings to determine whether MAP constituted a potential hazard to the public health. In step with the United Kingdom, Congress determined that there was sufficient scientific evidence to justify substantial funding in order to determine if MAP in milk constituted a public health hazard. But rather than awarding funding to the National Institutes of

Health or the Centers for Disease Control and Prevention, surprisingly, Congress gave stewardship of its implied mandate to USDA.

With what was ultimately over 90 million dollars at its disposal, USDA set about to explore addressing eradication of MAP within the production area.

In April of 2002, USDA-APHIS implemented the Uniform Program Standards for the Volunteer Bovine Johne's Disease Control Program and instituted a five year Johne's Disease Prevention Dairy Herd Demonstration Program.

Rather than addressing the elephant in the room, MAP as a public health hazard, USDA chose to do a test-and-cull demonstration program aimed at enhancing production economics. When it became apparent that a policy of identifying infected animals and removing them from the herd was neither economically feasible nor capable of eliminating MAP from infected herds, the massive demonstration project became simply an expensive data gathering vehicle that lost its scientific reason for being.

RECRUITMENT

My involvement with MAP and Crohn's disease began in 1969 on a cold January Saturday at Cross Creek, Florida.

After the organizers of the bass tournament had drawn for the pairing of partners, two individuals were left: J. Elliot Williams and I. Neither one of us had a boat, much less a bass boat. I had access to an electric trolling motor. Renting a boat and motor and having one person fish while the other held the trolling motor against the side of the boat, a friendship was born. Elliot won the tournament and I came in a respectable fifth.

Elliot had worked in various capacities as a laboratory technician and as a senior biological scientist at the University of Florida College of Veterinary Medicine.

About the time I left the University of Florida College of Medicine to become a professor at Creighton University School of Medicine, and ultimately an assistant dean, Elliot had begun working for a distinguished veterinary pathologist at the University of Florida College of Veterinary Medicine, Claus D. Buergelt. His research interests centered on *Mycobacterium avium* subspecies *paratuberculosis*. By virtue of his employment, Claus' interests became Elliot's. When it did not focus on fishing, our correspondence often involved Elliot's work in Claus' laboratory. In retrospect, he was slowly playing out the bait to me.

When you are not interested in a subject, you tend to be either a slow learner or what Italians term a "*capa dura*".

Exchanges concerning MAP did not graciously transcend the barriers of distance and time. When I finally got it, I got it. Veterinary medicine and that for humans were on a collision course from which there could be but two losers. MAP had the potential to be an incredible two headed dragon: the first, a threat to the nation's economy and the second, a threat to the public health.

While I was still at Creighton University School of Medicine, Elliot arranged for me to meet Professor Claus Buergelt.

Claus was then the longtime treasurer for the International Association for Paratuberculosis. Even though I was then recognized in Who's Who in Science and Technology as well as Medicine, co-founded both the U.S. and the International Infectious Disease Society for Obstetrics and Gynecology, and wrote the definitive text on the subject, these achievements bore little to no significance in the world of veterinary medicine or initially to Claus.

While previously at the University of Florida College of Medicine, I had created a virtual company, Infectious Diseases Incorporated (IDI) to capitalize on my knowledge about infectious diseases. IDI had functioned primarily as a research and educational resource for the pharmaceutical industry and the American College of Obstetricians and Gynecologists.

Once I became an assistant dean at Creighton, I had to farm out scientific ideas to colleagues at other institutions. I was literally rusting out. Having published well over a hundred peer-reviewed papers and a similar number in non-peer reviewed publications, there were but a few burning issues dealing with obstetrical or gynecological infectious diseases.

When the opportunity presented itself for possible early retirement, I took it. MAP offered me the opportunity to return to engineering bench research. In 2001, I started "a daring adventure with cows" (Helen Keller - "Life is a daring adventure or nothing").

Returning to Florida was a homecoming. Come football season, I bleed orange and blue. My four children had been born in Gainesville. Despite living in Omaha, Nebraska, I had kept my beach home in Cedar Key, some 60 miles due west of Gainesville. Gaining acceptance at the University of Florida College of Veterinary Medicine was facilitated by my prior employment at the University of Florida College of Medicine. The then Vice President of Medical Affairs, Gerald Schiebler's strong endorsement carried uncontestable weight. In 2001, Charles Courtney, Associate Dean for Research and Graduate Studies gave me a courtesy faculty appointment in the Department of Pathobiology at the University of Florida College of Veterinary Medicine as a Visiting Scientist. Later that year, a strategic partnership was signed between Infectious Diseases Incorporated and the College of Veterinary Medicine.

The initial passport into Dr. Buergelt's laboratory was Elliot's strong recommendation. Claus was true to his Germanic heritage. He was a strong believer in the law of gravity: translated, nothing defied that law, including innovative ideas.

The ultimate passport into Claus' laboratory was money. Years before, Doctor Schiebler had taught me that "Fiscal control is total control". The first seed money came from IDI. I penned the subsequent grants that became the fiscal underpinnings for Claus' laboratory.

Despite our divergent French and German heritages, in time Claus and I established a relationship of mutual respect. In the end, Claus would describe me to other veterinarians as the scientist from Mars. Two very special individuals, Jerry Davis and Maureen Davidson, along with Elliot, translated Martian into a living language for Claus.

A GARDEN OF WELL FERTILIZED WEEDS

*"A little bit of fertilizer benefits the garden of science,
but too much fertilizer stinks up the house of science".*

The garden of MAP was a mess. Creative investigative work into the immune response induced by MAP and genomic characterization of MAP had produced beautiful flowers. But, their presence tended to be overshadowed by a large number of "measurement papers" which, more often than not, lacked a governing hypothesis.

"Measurement without a hypothesis is not science".

Worse was the frequent advancement of a theory as scientific law that had not been substantiated by experimentation designed to challenge its premise.

When you are extended an invitation to live in someone else's conceptual house, you try to live by the house rules; so it was with paratuberculosis.

Explanation of the pathogenesis of MAP infection/Johne's disease had been constructed by Claus and the godfather of veterinary pathology, Robert Whitlock. Based upon primarily measurement observations, they had envisioned a three stage progression from infection to disease as being the natural history of MAP infection.

In stage one, the infected animal is asymptomatic. No detectable antibodies to MAP are present. Demonstration of the organism's presence is limited to the possible demonstration of MAP in feces. Stage two occurs months to years later. Antibodies to MAP are now demonstrable; however, the animal is still without clinical manifestation of diarrhea and weight loss. Stage three is characterized by multiple soft stools that progress to watery diarrhea and, in time, the death of the animal.

- **The following segment is technically dense. A lay reader may profit by passing over this section and proceeding to the heading: The Paratuberculosis Letter.**

The proposed natural history of MAP and, in particular, the long period of latency differed from that known for other pathogenic mycobacteria. Only *Mycobacterium leprae* had any overlapping features. My first instinct was to give my peers credence; but that became short lived.

The natural history of MAP infection/Johne's disease had been constructed using two tools: MAP recovery from feces and demonstration of antibodies to MAP. When examined closely, the tools and the conclusion derived from their use were found to be wanting.

Fecal recovery of MAP was stated to be the "gold standard" by which MAP infection was documented. While being highly specific for MAP, culture identification was notoriously insensitive. You could have a diseased animal with a high anti-MAP antibody titer and still not recover MAP from its stool. The obvious question was if you had a recovery system that failed to identify MAP in documented cases of infection/disease, how well did it function for animals with early, subclinical infection? The answer was, poorly.

Cow feces became a cesspool for poorly thought out ideas.

When feces contained large quantities of MAP, such animals were designated as "super shedders" and as such, were deemed to constitute a significant risk to their uninfected herd mates. When a fecal specimen grew out a certain number of MAP colonies, the significance of the observation and term were often transposed to the animal without a corresponding correlation to the animal's health status. Identification of being a super shedder was a potential passport to a premature exit from the herd and transportation to a slaughter house.

Unlike *M. bovis*, MAP grows *in vivo* in clumps, By virtue of its growth-pattern, the clump size variation and their distribution within a fecal specimen had the potential to be uneven. These facts should have alerted investigators to the potential that quantitative assessment of the growth of MAP from a fecal sample could be biased, not only by sample error, but by clump sizes within the fecal sample.

To investigate the potential for sample error, IDI teamed up with USDA officials in Florida. They facilitated access and use of specimens from USDA's Florida Johne's Disease Dairy Herd Demonstration Project.

The hypothesis was that sample errors existed within MAP fecal specimens. The experimental design to challenge the hypothesis was simple: have three different samples from the same fecal specimen tested by three diverging diagnostic tests done at different veterinary diagnostic laboratories. The participating laboratories were blinded as to the clinical status of the animals being sampled. Serum from each animal was sent to the State of Florida Veterinary Diagnostic Laboratory for the determination of whether anti-MAP antibodies was present.

Out of the 327 fecal samples analyzed, 22 animals were identified as heavy shedders. Ten fecal specimens lacked isolation confirmation by the two other tests. None of the animals had detectable anti-MAP antibodies in their blood.

Five of these animals had their blood retested from 8 to 14 months later. Again, no anti-MAP antibodies were identified.

This type of information began to put into question the natural history of MAP infection. In defense of the Buergelt-Whitlock postulate of the natural history of MAP, Whitlock advanced the idea that the transient fecal identification of MAP in the absence of anti-MAP antibodies was due to "pass through".

What was meant by pass through was that the animal ingested MAP, but the microbes did not attach to the mycobacterium receptor sites that line the entire gastrointestinal tract. That "pass through" attained acceptance in the veterinary literature was a tribute to the esteem with which Robert Whitlock was held by the veterinary community.

The real gold standard for the documentation of MAP infection was not fecal recovery, but rather the confirmation of infection at necropsy. Because of the difficulty in obtaining a large number of observations in order to achieve statistical significance, the gold standard was rarely used. But when it was used, necropsy-based data demonstrated that what was thought to be known about Johne's disease was distorted by literal smoke and mirrors.

In the United States, the two principle blood tests to determine the presence of MAP antibodies were HerdChek® and ParaChek®. Both these USDA certified tests set the standards against which every other MAP serological test was judged. When tested against the necropsy gold standard, these serum tests identified at best 30% of infected animals. At worst, McKenna and coworkers showed that commercial MAP ELISA tests detected only 6.8% - 8.8% of tissue positive cattle. In our published data, the correlation between the presence in animal feces and a positive commercial MAP ELISA test varied between 7.3% - 13.5%.

Beyond the marginal predictability of determining whether an animal was infected was the observation that HerdChek® and ParaChek® occasionally would produce test results that contradicted each other. The HerdChek® would identify a rare cow with Johne's disease as having specific anti-MAP antibodies and the ParaChek® would not and vice versa. The "Why?" was dismissed as laboratory error.

The why resided in the differences within the antigens embedded in the respective tests. In one case, the antigenic array was not derived from a proto-typical strain of MAP, but from *Mycobacterium* 18, a mycobacterium that was more like *Mycobacterium avium* than MAP. The two tests had identified mycobacterium strains that were closely interrelated yet distinct enough to cause a false-negative test.

Once IDI developed its first-generation MAP ELISA test and received USDA certification for its laboratory use, comparative tests were done.

Test sera were drawn from specimens obtained from the University of Florida's Demonstration Dairy Herd that Claus's veterinary diagnostic laboratory had been monitoring. Eighteen sera with known titer of antibodies were identified and retested using ParaChek®, HerdChek® and IDI's MAP ELISA test. Neither ParaChek® nor HerdChek® identified any of the low positive sera identified by our test; two and one respectively out of the six intermediate positive sera; and four and five out of the strongly positive sera.

To push what was becoming obvious a little further, cases, classical for Johne's disease, that still had samples of both serum and feces available were extracted from the archives of the College of Veterinary Medicine. The presence of a mycobacterium in the fecal specimen was confirmed using primers that could identify *Mycobacterium avium* (MAA)-like mycobacterium as well as MAP.

The corresponding serum samples were sent to the State of Florida's Veterinary Diagnostic Center and analyzed using the ParaChek® MAP ELISA test. The test done in Claus' laboratory identified six of the nine sera as containing anti-MAP antibodies. The ParaChek® test identified positive two sera as being positive. The test results were published in The Paratuberculosis Newsletter.

What was important was that, despite classical necropsy findings of Johne's disease having been present, neither of the MAP ELISA tests had completely identified the presence of MAP antibodies.

The inference was that these unidentified cases of necropsy confirmed Johne's disease were due to mycobacteria whose antigenic spectrum was not detected by the tests utilized.

USDA had made the internal decision that MAP was THE cause of Johne's disease and that mycobacteria, like the *Mycobacterium avium* complex and *Mycobacterium hominissuis,* were but environmental contaminants.

In MAP's evolution from *Mycobacterium avium* (MAA), one could argue for the existence of pathogenic mycobacteria that differed sufficiently in their genetic makeup so as to go undetected by MAP specific ELISA tests.

The challenge was to prove it. One of the earliest tests for the detection of MAP was called the agar immunodiffusion (AGID) test. The test consisted of pouring a small amount of agar into a small dish and letting it harden like Jell-O that has been left in the icebox too long. One then punches a central hole and one or more outer holes. The MAP antigens go into the central hole and the serum, which may or may not contain anti-MAP antibodies, is placed in the outer hole. Both the antigens and antibodies move towards each other. If they unite, a visible precipitation band forms.

The test has a 100% correlation with advanced systemic MAP disease. To Claus's everlasting credit, he continued to use this test when every other diagnostic veterinary laboratory had abandoned it.

The experimental design was simple. The study population was composed of Johne's diseased animals that, at necropsy, had had a positive AGID precipitation band. Their serum was then tested with our USDA certified MAP ELISA test. Of the 71 cases of Johne's disease with a positive AGID test, 12.7% of the animals lacked demonstrable anti-MAP antibodies.

Several cows demonstrated something not described in the literature, a second precipitation band. When queried about this observation, Claus said that it occasionally happened. The resultant question "why?" was addressed by gathering all the test results that had exhibited the double band phenomenon. The second band appeared only when the MAP ELISA titer was very high and would disappear when the titer dropped.

The first band had been presumed to identify the MAP specific antigen complex as used in the MAP ELISA tests. The fact that the first band could be demonstrated in Johne-diseased animals that lacked MAP antibodies indicated that the second band, and not the first band, were due to MAP specific antibodies.

Dare provided additional confirmation. She was a congenitally infected calf born to a Johne-diseased mother. Serial observations from birth through five months of age demonstrated that she eliminated her maternally acquired specific anti-MAP antibodies well before her AGID test became negative. That led to IDI's identification of a super mycobacterium antigen common to a number of different bovine pathogenic mycobacteria.

The next step did not require an experimental design. A current list of mycobacterium isolated from cattle by USDA over a two year period was obtained. A significant number of these isolates came from material forwarded from slaughter houses. Among the isolates were *M. hominissuis, M. avium* complex isolates and a rare *M. avium.*

Why USDA tenaciously held to MAP being THE cause of Johne's disease defied logic. In 2010, a friend handed me a copy of US patent No. 6,277,581 B1 dated August 21, 2001: Species Specific Genetic Identification of *Mycobacterium Paratuberculosis.* The patent's inventors were Jay Ellington and Judith Stabel of USDA.

When either USDA or the diagnostic tests manufacturers were asked, not what a positive HerdChek® or ParaChek® signified, but what a negative test meant, the answer was silence. If a HerdChek® or ParaChek® test did not demonstrate the presence of anti-MAP antibodies, the presumption to the person requesting the test was that the animal had not been infected by MAP.

The above data forced IDI to redesign the antigenic array of IDI's MAP ELISA test in order to better cover the genetic spectrum of MAP. The new test was used in a comparative study with ParaChek®'s MAP ELISA test. The study population consisted of sera from two separate dairy herds located across the road from each other.

One herd had been enrolled for four years in the USDA Florida Dairy Demonstration Project. When an animal tested positive in ParaChek's ® MAP ELISA test, it was culled. This herd had met USDA's designation of being MAP/Johne's disease free.

The other herd had had its animals tested. If a cow tested positive but looked good and was producing ample milk, she stayed within her milking group. This herd had had cows with clinical disease. The two herds constituted a comparative demonstration as to whether USDA's policy of test-and-cull eliminated MAP from dairy herds.

Sera from both herds were coded and then mixed together so that the person doing the test would have no knowledge as to which herd the serum specimen came from. The ParaChek® tests were done by the State of Florida Veterinary Diagnostic Laboratory.

Of the 27 sera obtained from the herd certified as being MAP-free, all 27 sera tested negative by the ParaChek® MAP ELISA test. Ten sera tested positive by Claus's laboratory.

Of the sera from the dairy known to have MAP diseased cows, out of the 23 sera analyzed, the ParaChek® ELISA system identified two as being positive and 10 as being suspicious. The IDI MAP ELISA test identified 15 out of the 23 sera as testing positive.

What distinguished the positive sera in the two dairy herds was the degree to which an individual cow's immune system had responded to MAP challenge. Removal of cows that tested positive in the ParaChek® MAP ELISA test did result in overall lower MAP titers within that herd. This data was published in The Paratuberculosis Newsletter.

The FUIDI #1 MAP ELISA test (FU= Florida University plus IDI = Infectious Diseases Incorporated) was incorporated into US Patents No. 8,008,033 B2, No. 8,143,012, and No. 8,366,173.

MAP VACCINES

Live and killed MAP vaccines have been shown to be effective in reducing the progression of MAP infection to disease form. What they have failed to do is interrupt the spread within the herd. The evolving paradigm is less about prevention of disease and more about limiting the amount of MAP entering into the human food chain.

The proposed newer vaccines are designed more to circumvent problems like cross reactivity with *M. bovis* or avoidance of granulomatous lesions at the site of vaccination. Rather than breaking new ground, the vaccines in development target the same objective in different wrappers.

Because MAP can be disseminated to other organs, a key question has been why the gastrointestinal tract is the sole site of manifested disease.

MAP is acquired through oral ingestion. In Johne's disease, the portal of infection and the target organ are one and the same. Unlike tuberculosis due to *Mycobacterium tuberculosis*, secondary redistribution of the organism to the target organ is not necessary. Yet MAP vaccines are administered systemically.

The effecter immune cells that need to be targeted reside within the submucosa. For a vaccine to be effective, it is theorized that the vaccine candidate has to:

1) be orally administered,

2) be attenuated, and

3) after inactivation, still bind to complimentary mycobacterium receptor sites.

The US Patent Office awarded IDI US patent No. 7,476,539 B1 which describes methodology that:

1) attenuates oral MAP vaccine candidates,

2) effects inactivation of the MAP oral vaccine candidates, and

3) documents the integrity of vaccine candidate's complementary receptor after inactivation.

COW #6142

The veterinary literature is uniform in its statement that "there is no cure for Johne's disease". That so-called scientific truth could have been embraced was it not for cow number 6142.

Number 6142 was a six year old Holstein cow with far advanced Johne's disease. Polymerase chain reaction (PCR) tests of milk and blood samples were repeatedly positive for MAP DNA. MAP had been isolated from fecal samples. When she had to go, she had to go. I watched a stream of liquid feces splatter against a wall some six feet away. What endeared her was the high titer of anti-MAP antibodies in her serum.

IDI purchased her from the University of Florida Demonstration Dairy Herd and had her relocated to a controlled research facility. The primary objective was to obtain a large amount of high tittered anti-MAP sera before her anticipated demise.

Normally, an animal in her condition would die within two to three weeks. In an attempt to delay her necropsy, cow numbered 6142 was placed on supplemental nutrition designed to enhance cell-mediated immunity. To our collective surprise, she decided that dying of diarrhea induced malnutrition was not an option that she liked.

Within ten days on the supplementation and stress reduction, her watery diarrhea converted to soft stools. After four months on supplementation, she gained over 200 kg.

Her MAP ELISA titer dropped to a near normal range. Her AGID tests become negative necropsy. At necropsy, the gastrointestinal tract exhibit no gross evidence of Johne's disease.

Microscopic examination of 34 microscopic slides of her gastrointestinal tract failed to identify any demonstrable MAP. With the exception of a rare granuloma in the corresponding lymph nodes, no evidence of MAP and its induced destructive change could be identified.

Having done her necropsy, Claus, unaware of what was being done to her, was so impressed that he published cow number 6142 as a case of spontaneous remission of Johne's disease.

In subsequent studies with diseased animals, the supplemented nutrition, now termed immunonutritional therapy, could usually terminate the watery diarrhea in seven to ten days and sustained the animal's life; but it did not impact on the totality of disease without concomitant stress reduction.

Cow number 6142 told the world that Johne's disease can be beneficially impacted by aggressive, monitored nutritional intervention, stress reduction and theoretically antimicrobial therapy.

Scientifically, cow number 6142 made an even more important contribution. When I reviewed her necropsy slides, I was stunned. In every one of the slides taken of her gastrointestinal tract, the area known as the lamina propria was crammed full of white blood cells called eosinophils. Eosinophils are involved in disease due to certain parasites. If I had not known cow number 6142's background history, based upon the histopathology, her diagnosis would have been idiopathic eosinophilic enteritis.

What cow number 6142 demonstrated is that the release of eosinophil-derived neurotoxins, enzymes and cationic proteins are instrumental in the end stage destruction of mycobacteria.

This hypothetical inference demanded proof. From the necropsy files of the University of Florida College of Veterinary Medicine, sequential cases of bovine Johne's disease necropsied by Claus were pulled. To establish the two study populations, slides of ileum were reviewed in order to identify the presence or absence of increased eosinophilia. For each case, the slides of ileum and a corresponding lymph node were analyzed to determine the amount of mycobacteria identifiable by special stains.

As inferred by cow number 6142, the presence of significant increase in the amount of eosinophils within the lamina propria inversely correlated with the amount of detectable MAP, in both small bowel and the draining lymph node.

In the veterinary pathology literature, two different types of Johne's disease are described: multibacillary Johne's disease in which many acid-fast bacilli are demonstrable and paucibacillary Johne's disease in which the number of acid-fast bacilli are markedly reduced. The explanation that had been advanced was that multibacillary and paucibacillary presentations reflected divergent host responses to MAP. What cow number 6142 revealed was that these two observations were not horizontal cuts through two divergent responses to infection, but rather a horizontal cut through various phases of the same infection.

If one is ever created, cow number 6142 needs to be enshrined in the Johne's disease Bovine Hall of Fame.

REVAMPING MAP'S
NATURAL HISTORY

The Buergelt-Whitlock theory of the pathogenesis of MAP infection/disease was embedded in the prevailing herd management schemas.

Rather than embrace it as a "scientific truth", we thought that it was, more probable than not, that the natural history of MAP infection paralleled that described for other pathogenic mycobacterium.

In the evolving MAP paradigm, the critical issue shifted from disease avoidance to the shedding of pathogenic mycobacteria into milk and milk products embedded in the human food supply. IDI's data as well as that of others had documented that subclinical MAP infection did not preclude the presence of MAP in milk. Of added concern was the presence of pathogenic mycobacteria identified by IS 1311 primers in the milk of cows that possessed no detectable MAP antibodies.

It had to be presumed that MAP acted very much like another mycobacterium, *M. tuberculosis* (the dominant cause of tuberculosis in humans). It was postulated that the majority of MAP challenged cows would develop a transient active infection from which the majority of these cows would recover. The key issue would be designing a way that would distinguish infected cows who had recovered from animals with still recent or active infection.

To challenge that hypothesis, IDI engineered a new MAP ELISA test (FUIDI # 2 MAP ELISA test) that increased the probability of identifying that infection was either active or of recent origin.

IDI tested 1,113 cows within USDA's Florida Johne's Disease Dairy Herd Demonstration Project. One hundred and ten cows had anti-MAP antibodies as identified by the FUIDI #2 MAP ELISA test. Nine of these cows had levels consistent with advanced disease. Another six cows had titers consistent with either evolving or receding significant MAP infection.

Fourteen months later, 551 of the original 1,113 cows were available for re-analysis. Of the original 91 infected cows, 54 were available for retesting, 45 cows no long tested positive for active infection. Eight cows had serological evidence of continuing infection and two had progressed to very active infection/disease status. What was most impressive was that, of the 540 cows that had previously test negative, fourteen months later, 18.9% of these cows now had evidence of acute infection.

IDI patented the FUIDI Herd Management Schema whose foundations centered on the demonstrated fact that in most cases of bovine MAP infection, host immunity can abort MAP's continued replication.

The FUIDI Herd Management Schema was designed to be more than a tool by which producers could reduce losses sustained from decreased milk production, lower cow fertility, reduction in slaughter weight and increase herd immunity to environmental mycobacterium challenges. Its ultimate purpose was to decrease the amount of MAP in milk, cheeses, baby formula and other milk-based foods.

A POORLY TILLED GARDEN

In 2012, OIE contemplated throwing in the towel. MAP had become so prevalent among milk producing animals that it proposed removing paratuberculosis as a disease entity from the Terrestrial Animal Health Code ***"because MAP infection is so widespread, continued recognition of MAP as an animal pathogen would only cause economic losses through the restrictions in international animal trade".***

The decision by USDA to allow the MAP ELISA tests to be a statement of probability rather than a valid measurement of the amount of antibody present, permitted infectious cows to be transported across state lines and national borders with relative ease contrary to the Animal Health Protection Act (7 U.S.C. 8301 *et seq.*).

In 2002, USDA had estimated that between 20-30% of US dairy herds contained one or more MAP infected/diseased animals. By 2007, the number had increased to 70%. By 2015, a number between 90 and 100% might well be correct.

Traditionally, animal health quality of assurance is addressed by the animal's health certificate. The language in many state health certificates tends to minimize any requirement that the animal be free of underlying infectious diseases. The certificates merely require that the certificate be signed by a veterinarian attesting to the apparent absence of any contagious or otherwise transmissible disease. The Code of Federal Regulations (9 CFR, chapter 1 subchapter C) specifically restricts the interstate movement of MAP-infected animals except to recognized slaughter establishments for processing. Its language prohibits or restricts the interstate movement of livestock that have, or have been exposed to Johne's disease. Documentation of infection and/or disease is contingent upon voluntary testing, that, if done, it would be economically counter-productive for producers.

The Wisconsin Implied Warranty law stipulates that cattle to be sold are guaranteed to be MAP-free, unless sellers provide a written retraction of this guarantee at the time of the sale.

In 2008, USDA unveiled its National Johne's Disease Control Program Strategic Plan that identified but three specific goals:

- Reduce the prevalence of MAP/Johne's disease in the national herd
- Reduce the impact of Johne's disease on individual herds
- Reduce the risk of introducing Johne's disease to uninfected herds

This strategic plan would later be referred to in private as USDA's "closing the barn door after the cows had left strategic program".

USDA's prior decision that allowed MAP ELISA tests to basically be a statement of probability rather than a valid measurement of the amount of antibody undermined two of its three mission objectives.

The decision by USDA not to require a statement as to an animal's MAP status has undermined its avowed intent to prevent dissemination of MAP into uninfected herds. By not requiring a statement as to whether an animal is or is not infected by MAP on its health certificate, cows have been, and are being, shipped across state and even national borders. The net result has been not only the introduction of infected animals into previously uninfected herds, but, an overall increasing prevalence of MAP infection in the national herds.

From 2001 through 2014, what USDA has effectively done was to take a manageable problem and make it into one of colossal proportions. Today, it is more probable than not, that no large dairy operation in the United States is free of MAP infected cows and that the number of infected animals is significant.

Gilles R. G. Monif M.D.

THE PARATUBERCULOSIS
NEWSLETTER

After publishing two scientific papers, Claus suggested that I join The International Association for Paratuberculosis. The organization's official publication is The Paratuberculosis Newsletter. Its editorial board had been composed of veterinarians primarily from the University of Minnesota and the University of Wisconsin.

When Congress's concerns about MAP materialized into the funding of its mandate, the American contingent within the International Paratuberculosis Association shifted their focus to their newly created society, the Johne's Disease Interdisciplinary Program (JDIP). JDIP convinced USDA to allow it to be the principal conduit through which MAP research would be funded. The governors of JDIP then set out to unite all in the scientific community involved with MAP under their banner. The carrot held out was possible funding. Creating JDIP had the potential to be a brilliant move, had it been properly implemented. Being the avowed thought leaders, members of JDIP often constituted the principle reviewers for U.S. veterinary journals.

With most of the U.S. researchers' overriding commitment to JDIP, their participation in The Paratuberculosis Newsletter effectively disappeared. The net result was that the informational content of The Paratuberculosis Newsletter became more limited. The responsibility for the scientific integrity of The Paratuberculosis Newsletter fell to the Europeans. Soren Nielsen, a Danish veterinarian, took on the vacated position of editor.

In his resignation speech, the president of the International Association for Paratuberculosis, Michael Collins published the following: "*In spite of the fundamental importance of the zoonosis question, it is getting limited funding and therefore limited attention. Agriculture- related funding organizations do not consider the zoonosis question their funding responsibility; in fact they may feel it is not in their best interest to discover that M. paratuberculosis is a zoonotic pathogen. Medical, food and water research funding organizations, generally do not fund research on animal diseases and seem to be waiting for someone else to decide that M. paratuberculosis is a zoonotic agent before investing in research on this pathogen. And so, year by year and colloquium after colloquium, we scientists produce data and exchange information on research questions, related to the veterinary concerns and not the zoonotic question.*"

Nature abhors a vacuum. The resultant void created the opportunity for IDI to disseminate information without revealing information that could invalidate the patentability of its intellectual properties. The negative by-product was a limitation on the information that it could freely disseminate or publish in peer reviewed journals.

To expand dialogue and content within The Paratuberculosis Newsletter, IDI began providing a number of small fragments of research based data that did not impinge upon its intellectual properties.

Gilles R. G. Monif M.D.

"A procedure to assist in the identification of slow growing mycobacterium from slants";

"Duration of bovine maternally acquired antibodies to Mycobacterium avium subspecies paratuberculosis: A case study";

Use of blotted tissue impressions for the rapid PCR identification of Mycobacterium avium subspecies paratuberculosis";

"Persistent bovine fecal MAP shedding in the first month of life;
Once an academic footprint had been created, IDI began an educational campaign directed at preparing milk producers and milk-based manufacturers as how to mitigate the potential that MAP and Crohn's disease were more than just interconnected.

The September 2008 issue contained a debate paper entitled *"What if: A contrarian's questioning of the natural history of bovine infection due to Mycobacterium avium subspecies paratuberculosis."* The article drew no response, but the idea had its public debut.

In December 2008, the discussion introduced centered on the lack of MAP certification of cattle being sold. Its conclusion statement stated. *"Unless otherwise clearly stated, Certificates of Health for dairy cows need to have the words, buyer beware added".*

In order to stabilize the price of milk, in 2009, the National Milk Producer Federation Cooperative instituted a policy of reducing herd size by paying producers slaughter price for the cows removed from production. The comments in the September issue described the opportunity to improve herd quality through selective testing for MAP and animal slaughter selection based upon risk.

The December article, *'An Ounce of Prevention is Worth More than a Pound of Cure"*, again centered on animal certificates of health. Beef and dairy producers in Texas had a habit of reaching down into Mexico and buying cattle on the cheap. The problem was that many herds had not only paratuberculosis but also bovine tuberculosis.

Mexico exports one million cattle annually to the United States. Based upon APHIS's own statistics, 75% of bovine tuberculosis (*M. bovis*) detected through sometimes sporadic slaughter surveillance originated in Mexico. In 2009, chronic draught conditions had forced relocation of cattle to a large number of dairy and beef states. Slaughter identification was detection after the fact and more importantly, after infected animals had been shipped out of the area. The problem that USDA was now having with *M. bovis* was a marker for the undetected dissemination of MAP throughout the U.S. dairy and beef herds.

The March 2010 contribution, *"When is Mycobacterium Avium Sub- species Paratuberculosis Mycobacterium Avium Variant and When is Mycobacterium Avium Mycobacterium Avium subspecies Paratuberculosis?"* was an attempt to bring back into focus that Johne's disease was not always caused by just MAP.

Gilles R. G. Monif M.D.

This editorial opinion was a partial restatement of an article published in the March 2009, "*The Difference between an A and The* (cause of Johne's disease), and the March 2011 Paratuberculosis Newsletter, "*Are Mycobacterium avium subspecies avium and Mycobacterium avium complex pathogens?*"

THE 10TH INTERNATIONAL COLLOQUIUM ON PARATUBERCULOSIS

Minneapolis MN October 28th, 2010

The 10th International Colloquium on Paratuberculosis (ICP) was chosen to present IDI's versions of errors-up-to date/ scientific truths. In collaboration with our colleagues from the University of Florida College of Veterinary Medicine and Purdue University School of Veterinary Medicine, IDI submitted eight presentations that spanned everything from diagnostic immunology to herd epidemiology.

Being hosted by JDIP, our papers could not crack a pre-selected program agenda. In retrospect that worked to our advantage. The poster presentations worked in banding together contrarian investigators.

With poster presentations, one of the investigators would stand in front of large five foot by six foot posters and discuss the embedded data with interested parties. It is thus that we established contact with Ivo Pavlik and Eiichi Momotani among others.

Ivo Pavlik had been chosen to be one of the ICP's keynote speakers. He and Karel Hruska had just published a major text on MAP.

In a world long on intelligence, the creativity of a scientist is more in the question/hypothesis being asked, than the answered attained. The epidemiological and scientific studies carried out at the Veterinary Research Institute of the Czech Republic functioned at a high level in terms of scientific integrity and creativity. Professor Pavlik's work had elegantly documented the presence of MAP within infant formula derived from seven different countries.

Professor Eiichi Momotani was the director of Japanese Society for Paratuberculosis. Professor Momotani had had a central role in formulation of Japan's Act on Domestic Animal Infectious Disease Control as it related to MAP. In one of his publications, he had demonstrated the ability of MAP antigen to cause full thickness enteritis in mice (http:www.springerplus.com/content/pdf/2193-1801-47.pdf).

In subsequent correspondence, he expressed his concern about the US's lack of control over paratuberculosis, given its theorized effect upon Japan. He had found that the powdered milk used in the formulation of infant formula sold in Japan was imported primarily from the United States. In 2011, Japan had imported 5,016,451 kg of butter and 21, 424,350 kg of other dairy products. Previously, the Japanese health authorities had documented that 54% of MAP infected/diseased cows imported into Japan came from the United States.

Because the Japanese Ministry of Agriculture, Forestry and Fisheries looked to OIE for leadership and OIE's position mirrored that of USDA, Professor Momotani had been under increasing pressure to not challenge the Ministry's position with respect to MAP.

A featured component of the 10th ICP was a debate between Herbert J. Van Kruininger, a senior veterinary pathologist, and Thomas J. Bull from Hermon-Taylor's group on whether or not MAP'was causally related to Crohn's disease.

In the mid-1980s and early 1990s, Van Kruiningen had been actively involved with the causative hypothesis. Chiodini had co-published several papers with him in the mid-1980s. In a 1984 article, using a crude antigen derived from a MAP strain obtained from an individual with Crohn's disease, Thayer, Coutz, Chiodini, Van Kruiningen and Merkal demonstrated that individuals with Crohn's disease had a statistically significant increase in anti-MAP antibodies. In 1991, Van Kruiningen co-authored a paper that reaffirmed that MAP could cross species barriers. A MAP isolate of human derivation has been shown to produce experimental disease in chicken. Now, more than a decade later, he was arguing against his earlier scientific leanings. The inability to culture MAP from individuals with Crohn's disease using technology that achieved MAP from animals with Johne's disease, the inability to demonstrate the presence of MAP using special stains within diseased tissues, contradicting serological findings with human sera and the inability of some investigators to reduplicate Naser's earlier work had converted Van Kruiningen into a fervent champion of the hypothesis' denial.

The question and answer period was not kind to Van Kruiningen. Studies cited in defense of his position often had flawed methodology. The failure to incorporate the innovations in diagnostic technology had left him stuck in a decade behind the prevailing state of the art.

Bull presented a composite of the work from Hermon-Taylor's group as it related to the technology required to demonstrate the presence of MAP. The inability of special stains to demonstrate the presence of MAP was due to the loss of its outer wall. Recovery of MAP requires special media that address MAP's existence as a spheroclast.

Before he left, Tom Bull placed a video copy of his presentation on IDI's web site (www. ismilksafe.org).

Kruiningen's arguments had some footing. Where he erred was in the ultimate interpretation of the data. What both debaters had documented is that, if MAP caused Crohn's disease, it did so by a mechanism different from that used by it to cause Johne's disease.

Bull's documentation of the positive correlation between tissue fixation of MAP DNA and disease left the causality issue clearly on the table of probability. The need was to answer the question of how.

After the debate, Kruiningen sought me out. To my literal amazement, he thanked me for comments that had been delivered with asbestos gloves: an act that spoke of character.

In 1999, Herbert J. Kruiningen published his presentation in the Journal of Inflammatory Bowel Disease (Kruiningen, H. J. Lack of support for a common etiology in Johne's disease of animals and Crohn's disease in humans. Inflamm. Bowel Dis. 1999; 5:183-91).

This article continues to have a life of its own. When pushed, this is the summary article advanced by FDA in defense of its position of silence.

Organized meetings of peers at any meeting become a place where politics play out. At the lunch recess between sessions, I asked Robert Whitlock to join me and discuss "pass through". As we walked out of the building, I saw a veterinarian from Thailand bow his head as a sign of respect as Professor Whitlock walked by. Robert Whitlock had been Claus' teacher and as such, he was personified as being holy ground to Claus and a vast number of veterinary pathologists. Such adulation had permitted his words to be unchallenged gospel, but at a price that had been costly in terms of advancing scientific knowledge.

At the end of the 10th ICP, Robert Whitlock and Claus Buergelt were honored for their lifelong service to the International Association for Paratuberculosis.

Politics isn't always about differences of opinion or acquiring brown nose status. There is often a darker side. The real "educational event" of the 10th ICP occurred in one of USDA's semi-closed session. Prionic (the manufacturers of ParaChek®) petitioned USDA to have their test and laboratory become the reference against which all laboratory certification MAP ELISA tests would be judged. It was fascinating to listen to a fox petitioning to be the keeper of the hen house.

When no meaningful objection was forthcoming from USDA, Michael Collins and the representative of IDDEX (manufacturer and distributor of HerdChek®) turned the prevailing sentiment in the other direction. Test certification responsibility remained with USDA.

MAP AND CROHN'S DISEASE FROM A MEDICAL PERSPECTIVE

While the non-PhD part of veterinary medicine was focused on feces and other biological fluids, the world of human medicine involved with humans was penning a strong circumstantial case for an etiological connection between MAP and Crohn's disease.

Ghadiali et al. documented that the human MAP isolates exhibited similar polymorphic locus patterns to animal MAP isolates, making it, more probable than not, that MAP isolates cultured from human beings could produce disease in susceptible animals. Other investigators have documented that MAP isolates cross species lines with relative ease. A goat or sheep MAP isolate can infect cattle and vice versa.

Naser et al. cultured MAP from the blood of 50% of patients with Crohn's disease, 22% of patients with ulcerative colitis and 0% of individuals without inflammatory bowel disease. His finding was of immense scientific significance; yet Naser was basically shunned by the world of veterinary medicine. In time, federal funding for his research vaporized.

Sechi et al. identified MAP DNA in 83.3% of the biopsies from patients with Crohn's Disease and 10.3% of control patients. Other investigators including Autschback et al. and Bull et al. confirmed the positive correlation between MAP and diseased gastrointestinal tissue from individuals afflicted with Crohn's disease. The positive correlation between the demonstration of MAP within diseased gastrointestinal tissue from Crohn's disease-afflicted individuals was but inferential.

A "scientific truth" must account for the exceptions. The presence of MAP in tissue from individuals without Crohn's disease required explanation

The explanation advanced was that Crohn's disease was but the pinnacle of MAP infection. Scana et al. presented evidence incriminating MAP as an etiological component of "irritable bowel syndrome" in humans. What was emerging was the inference that human MAP infection had a spectrum of possible outcomes ranging from asymptomatic subclinical infection, a slight increase in the number of bowel movements a day, irritable bowel disease, to Crohn's disease.

By 2008, sufficient evidence existed that the American Academy of Microbiologists published its report on *Mycobacterium avium paratuberculosis*: Infrequent Human Pathogen or Public Health Threat. The executive summary states, "*the association of MAP and CD (Crohn's disease) is no longer in question. **The critical issue today is not whether MAP is associated with CD, but whether MAP causes CD or is only incidentally present.**"

In 2009, three independent diagnostic laboratories (Michael T. Collins of the University of Wisconsin, Saleh A. Naser of the University of Central Florida, and Jack Crawford of the CDC tested blood from 58 individuals. Viable MAP was detected in 22 out of 40 with inflammatory bowel disease (20 with Crohn's disease and 20 with ulcerative colitis) and 4 of 18 subjects without inflammatory bowel disease. Two of the diagnostic centers detected MAP in 41% of the blood from individuals with inflammatory bowel disease and from 0% in the "control blood samples. In four cases, MAP was isolated from the blood of individuals without Crohn's disease. Their findings were subsequently confirmed by Juste and co-workers.

The isolation of a microbe from blood conclusively documents that an individual is infected by that organism. Rather than undermining the presumption of causality, the finding of systemically infected healthy humans among the study controls speaks to the probability that MAP had achieved a significant penetration into the population from which the control subjects were drawn. With at very least 2% of the milk that human consume containing viable MAP organisms and with MAP potentially being in powdered milk and milk based foods, particularly soft cheeses, it becomes a question of time and diet as to whether or not one becomes infected. Diet and age define the probability of an individual being infected.

What has been well documented is that milk, cheeses, and infant formula have the potential to be adulterated by a bovine pathogen, *Mycobacterium avium* subspecies *paratuberculosis* (MAP). In 2007, the National Animal Health Monitoring System study of 515 dairy farms identified the fact that 31.2% of the participating dairy farms had bulk tank milk positive for MAP DNA. MAP in concentrations from 48 to 32,500 live organisms per gram of powdered infant milk was found in 35% of 51 investigated samples. MAP DNA was detected in 4.2% to 31.7% of cheeses tested. In 2005, 49%

of 51 brands of baby formula manufactured by 10 different producers in seven different countries were demonstrated to contain MAP DNA. What these figures are in 2015 is open to speculation.

Mycobacterium receptors line the gastrointestinal tract. Oral ingestion of viable MAP equates with infection. Mycobacterium infection/disease each involve a phase in which the organism is in the blood stream. The presence of MAP in the blood of control subjects speaks the unintended exposure of a substantial segment of the U.S. population to MAP. In the latter studies, selection of control subjects had encompassed an occasional individual with active infection.

Part II

SINNING BY SILENCE

"To sin by silence when men should cry out, makes cowards of men."

Abraham Lincoln

SILENCE

In the United States, the veterinary response to MAP as a public hazard, much less the cause of irritable bowel syndrome (IBS), had but a muted voice. The proposed relationship between MAP and Crohn's disease would occasionally get lip service in the introduction of a paper. The topic was rarely revisited in the discussion of the significance of authors' findings. Lack of conclusive scientific proof would, more often than not, be cited as the rational for not pursuing in discussions of any depth.

Tobacco being the cause of lung cancer is a medical "scientific truth". That "truth" was not based upon absolute proof, but allegedly became accepted by government agencies when the insurance lobby demonstrated that the costs embedded in cancer exceeded the revenue stream, directly or indirectly, derived from tobacco. Whether that story is confabulation or not, the fact remains that the causation link between tobacco and cancer rests on something other than absolute proof.

When you want something done, you seek out the person in charge. In today's world, that person is called the CEO (Chief Executive Officer).

The topic proposed to industry was preserving the economical integrity of the dairy industry. The letter's last line stated: "For anything to work, it must obviously come from industry".

The possibility that, based upon the preponderance of credible scientific evidence, the potential presence of MAP in milk constituted a public health hazard should have been sufficient to penetrate industry's imposed shield of silence. Despite a number of attempts, no response was forth coming.

Persisting further, more likely than not, would invite retribution. What the Cattlemen's Association did to Oprah Winfrey had served as notice to the world of the virtue of sinning by silence.

My first attempt to publish in a U.S. veterinary journal a paper that challenged the prevailing dogma turned out to be an interesting exercise. I had a reviewer who did not believe anything that was not already proven. "The data was inconsistent with other publications".

Since one robin doesn't herald spring, the decision was made to test whether one was dealing with "bright men who were faking it or idiots who meant it." The instrument chosen was a Letter to the Editor. The integrity of any journal resides with its editor. The topic chosen was based on observations whose scientific validity was beyond scientific challenge.

Crafting the prevailing data into a coherent statement of facts in 300 words or less was analogous to fitting a size six document into a size two dress.

Gilles R. G. Monif M.D.

LETTER TO AN EDITOR

Failed Goals within the
National Johne's Disease Control Program

The 2008 National Johne's Disease Control Program Strategic Plan has failed in meeting two of the three of its stated objectives: reducing the prevalence of MAP/Johne's disease in the national herd and reducing the risk of introducing Johne's disease to uninfected herds (1)

The current commercial MAP ELISA tests measure anti-MAP antibodies, but the interpretation of a positive test is predicated on the identification of a level of antibody that predicts a high probability of a progression of MAP infection to overt enteritis or confirmation of disease. A negative commercial MAP ELISA test does not address the issue of whether or not a given animal is or ever has been infected by MAP. The decision by USDA to have the MAP ELISA tests represent a statement of probability rather than an accurate statement of the amount of antibody present has permitted infectious cows to be transported across state lines and national borders with relative impunity. The net result is not only the introduction of infected animals into uninfected herds, but an overall increased prevalence of MAP infection in the national herds. In 2007, an estimated 70% of U.S. dairy herds contained one or more infected animals (2).

The Japanese approach to containing MAP is embodied in its Act on Domestic Animal Infectious Disease Control. After 1998, every Japanese dairy farm is examined for MAP every five years. Imported cattle are subjected to quarantine in which they are screened using a MAP ELISA test, fecal bacterial culture, PCR analysis for fecal MAP DNA, and Johnin skin test. Fifty-four percent of diseased animals detected by the Japanese Animal Quarantine Service came from the United States (3).

The number of infectious cows shipped from the United States that escaped serological detection is open to speculation.

Gilles R.G. Monif, M.D.
Infectious Diseases Incorporated

References*

- *Schwartz A.: National Johne's Disease Control Program Strategic Plan. October 23, 2008. Page 1*

- USDA-APHIS Johne's Disease in U.S. Dairies 1991-2007. http://nahms.aphis.usda.gov/dairy http://aphis.usda.gov/dairy/dairy07/dairyJohnes.pdf.2007

- *Eiichi M.2012. Epidemiological situation and control strategies for paratuberculosis in Japan. Japanese J. Vet. Res. 60:19-29*

- (Publication of references at the discretion of editor – 300 word limit)

The rejection came directly from the Editor. What was unique was his comment that the editorial was "a thinly veiled advertisement of IDI"

A reviewer can lack knowledge. An editor of an influential journal has the right to disavow his duty to disseminate knowledge. Making an unprofessional remark became an invitation to a pointed discussion.

Dear_____;

"I was disappointed by your rejection of my letter to the editor. To present a case in 300 words or less, effectively limits citing the documentation in the literature. As an editor of a scientific journal, you would have had merely to read the manufacturer's product material to confirm an absence of any explanation as to the significance of a negative MAP ELISA test. The literature is overburdened with articles documenting the inability of the various certified MAP ELISA tests to achieve a reasonable correspondence between serological test results and culture data and/or slaughter observations. More simply put, the current negative MAP ELISA test results do not address the issue of whether an animal has had prior antigenic processing of MAP antigen (infection) and more importantly whether or not the animal is infectious. This is a subject very worthy of public scientific debate, i.e. an editorial debate. I would be more than willing to offer one side of the debate. I would be impressed if you would be able to find someone in USDA willing to debate in open forum the validity of a negative MAP ELISA test."

"I went to great lengths not to bring into focus any of IDI's work, expressively to avoid accusation of bias or as you chose to phrase it "thinly veiled advertisement of IDI". If my association with IDI is a concern for you, that could have been handled simply by you deleting my affiliation with IDI. The content of that editorial letter has nothing to do with IDI and everything to do with USDA and the consequences of their actions. Had I not clearly identified my association with IDI that would have been contrary to the policy of disclosure. The letter was an observation confirmable by anyone with reasonable knowledge of the literature."

"As far as advertisement of myself, I have no need. I am a nationally and internationally recognized researcher and leader in the area of infectious diseases as they adversely affect women and their unborn babies. More precisely I have published well over a hundred articles in peer reviewed medical journals, co-founded both the Infectious Disease Society for Infectious Diseases in Obstetrics and Gynecology and its internal counterpart, was the special interest consultant for the American College of Obstetricians and Gynecologist for over a decade, wrote the definitive text book on OB/GYN infection (currently in its sixth edition), was instrumental in developing CDC's change of position on two key infectious disease issues affecting women, etc., etc."

"IDI is a medical education/research entity founded in 1973. Why is a medical research entity involving itself into veterinary business? The answer is simply that MAP is a zoonotic pathogen that, like *M. bovis* in milk, appears to constitute a public health hazard. The bottom line is "a risk is a risk and must be addressed"; however, given the political power of the lobbyist of organizations like the _____ and the _____, open debate is being held hostage until means are attained that will assure the welfare of the dairy and milk related industries. In the meantime, everyone is asked "*to sin by silence when men should cry out makes cowards of men* (A. Lincoln)".

"Shortly, IDI expects to be announcing its schema that may allow the majority of infected cows to remain in production while decreasing the amount of MAP entering the human food supply. But IDI can do nothing about the spread of MAP into uninfected herds or decreasing the prevalence of MAP within a given herd. What was a containable problem in the late 1990s is now out of control."

To quote T. Roosevelt: "*When a decision is required, the best decision is to do the right thing. The next best decision is to do the wrong thing. The worst decision is to do nothing.*" Doing nothing has prevailed.

"If your ego is a little bruised, the easy thing will be to put this e-mail in a circular file. Perhaps a better course of action would be to forgive me for my aggressive response and have us work together for a better future outcome for the dairy industry."

Sincerely,
Gilles R. G. Monif, M.D.
President, IDI

Dear Dr. Gilles R. G. Monif:

Thank you for your e-mail. You are welcome to submit your research to Journal of for consideration as a published research article. If you are so inclined, submit it through normal channels. In glancing at your attachment, I note that you will need to conform to the guidelines for authors. Also, in the submission process, you will have the opportunity to suggest reviewers. In terms of guidelines, the short communication guidelines may be most consistent with your intent.

Sincerely,

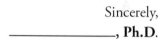_____, **Ph.D**.

The publications of Naser, Hermon-Taylor, Greenstein, Soren, Plavik, Hruska, among others, had published in primarily non-U.S. veterinary journals. When the sharing of research data permitted, IDI's submissions went across the pond or to St. Elsewhere.

Gilles R. G. Monif M.D.

THE HRUSKA POSTULATE

Hruska K., Slama J., Kralik P., Pavlik I. *Mycobacterium avium* subsp. *paratuberculosis* in powdered milk: F57 competitive real time PCR: Veterinarni Medicina 2011; 226-230 http://vri.cs/docs/vetmed/56-5-226.pdf

Hruska K., Pavlik: Crohn's disease and related inflammatory diseases: from a single hypothesis to one "superhypothesis." Veterinarni Medicina 2014; 59-583-630 http://vri.cs/docs/vetmed/59-12-583.pdf

The Veterinary Research Institute at Brno in the Czech Republic was the intellectual powerhouse within the world of veterinary medicine. Through its Centaur Global Network Information (CGNI), Karel Hruska compiled and disseminated, on a monthly basis, comprehensive lists of abstracts on various veterinary infectious disease topics. Information is power. This sharing of knowledge and the spirit with which it was done prompted me to contact Professor Karel Hruska.

In response to my email, on August 12, 2012, Professor Karel Hruska agreed to open a dialogue about collaborative research dealing with MAP. We were bonded by a mutual disdain for the buck-passing empty phrase, "Crohn's disease and MAP linkage is still unproven".

When Karel explained to me what I now term the **Hruska Postulate**, the limitations of my approach to addressing the Crohn's disease epidemic became embarrassingly apparent.

Therapies capable of producing a transient remission of Crohn's disease symptomolgy share one common documented factor: impairment of the effector arm of the immune system or neutralizing the cytokine, tumor necrosis factor-alpha.

While I had been wading through cow shit, Karel Hruska had distanced himself from the prevailing bullshit.

Put into simplistic terms, the Hruska Postulate argues that Crohn's disease is an immune induced disease caused by the loss of mucosal loss of tolerance to MAP's antigenic array.

What Crohn's disease is not is an autoimmune disease. In an immune mediated disease, the human body is responding to a specific set of antigens. In the case of Crohn's disease, the antigens are those of *Mycobacterium avium* subspecies *paratuberculosis*. The wall of MAP contains a glycopeptides, muramyl dipeptid (MDP) which exerts a powerful polyclonal immunostimulatory effect on lymphocytes and macrophages.

In constructing the postulate, Karel looked to experiments in nature for guidance. For him, natural experiments were infinitely more creative than anything anyone can dream up in the laboratory. Three sets of these natural experiments served as cornerstones for the Hruska Postulate.

I. Iceland's physical isolation made it an ideal epidemiological laboratory. Prior to the German "co-habitation" of Iceland, the disease caused by MAP in domestic animals had been undetected. In 1933, the Germans brought sheep to Iceland, some of which were infected by this organism. With time, MAP disease became epidemic in sheep and eventually in cattle. The incidence of Crohn's disease in Iceland from 1950-1959 was 0.4 cases per 100,000 individuals per year; from 1960-1969 0.9; from 1970-1979 3.1; from 1980-1989 3.11; and from 1990-1995 5.6.

II. World War II and then the Iron Curtain had isolated the **Czech Republic** from the world. Prior to1990, MAP infection and paratuberculosis were virtually unknown in milking herds within the Czech Republic. Economic hardships forced most mothers to breast feed their babies. Following the crumbling of the Iron Curtain, some 30,000 heifers were imported from countries whose herds contained animals with paratuberculosis. As the local economy improved, women began abandoning breast feeding in favor of milk or infant formula. Initially, infant formula was produced from local herds; however, the single local producer was bought by an international company and local production was stopped. The domestic product was replaced by imported formula. In 2005, it was demonstrated that 49% of 51 brands of baby formula manufactured by 10 different producers in seven different countries contained the DNA of MAP. Between 1995 and 2004, the incidence of Crohn's disease in the Czech Republic increased 4.5 fold among 0-19 year olds and 6.5 fold in 65+ year old individuals.

Just as in the **United States,** the dissemination of MAP among the milk producing animals had been the prerequisite for the initiation of the Icelandic and the Czech Republic's Crohn's disease epidemic.

In developing countries, the need for MAP dissemination among its milk-producing animals prior to the onset epidemics of Crohn's disease has been theoretically circumvented by the marketing of infant formula in lieu of breast feeding. The global market of infant formula has made baby food and dairy products potentially containing MAP accessible to the countries without MAP's dissemination within their milk-producing animals.

III. Protective Effect of Breast Feeding:

Within the Czech Republic's experiment in nature, there existed an embedded control subpopulation, Roma (gypsies). Breast feeding is culturally based among Roma women. Unlike their Czech counterparts, Roma women were much slower to adopt change. The rate of Crohn's disease among Roma has persistently been half the incidence of the rest of the Czech population.

The hypothesis of protection conferred by breast feeding is supported by observations of lower incidence of Crohn's disease in Canadian Indians, Maoris in New Zealand, Arab residents in Israel, the Gypsy population in Hungary and residents with a lower social status in many countries. The one common attribute for these ethnic or social groups is that breast feeding is practiced and newborns are less frequently fed infant formula.

Six retrospective studies assessing risk factors for the development of Crohn's have universally documented that breast feeding confers a protective effect against the future development of Crohn's disease.

The protective effect of breast feeding identifies a time frame in which loss of mucosal tolerance to MAP would have had to occur. Superimposition of the epidemiological studies that document the protective effect of breast feeding and the enhanced virulence of intra-cellular pathogens for newborn infants further defines the mechanism by which newborn MAP infection can translates years later, into Crohn's disease.

IV. Immune System Immaturity:

Very young animals do not handle challenges by intracellular pathogens, specifically those engendered by viruses and mycobacteria effectively.

In animals with intact immune systems, viral and mycobacterium replication are terminated by cell-mediated immunity. Thereafter, the organisms persist for an extended period of time within the host. DNA viruses such as the varicella-zoster virus (chickenpox/ shingles), the cytomegaloviruses, the Herpes simplex virus, and *Mycobacterium tuberculosis* have the very real potential for reactivation. The organisms escape immune containment and again induce disease.

Infection of fetuses and babies in the neonatal period (the first thirty days) by selected RNA and DNA viruses results in widespread systemic disease. If the baby lives, the residual damage usually results in lifelong disabilities. The same infections acquired after the second or third month of life usually result in relatively minimal clinical disease, if any.

Unlike extracellular pathogens (bacteria), intracellular viruses and mycobacteria, undergo a process termed "immune capture" in which isolation of the organism is no longer recoverable despite having continued immunological presence. Stimulation of a species specific humeral immunity continues. In the early 1940s, an epidemic caused by the rubella virus occurred on a remote island off the coast of Alaska. Thirty years later, a second epidemic occurred. Those who were born following the initial epidemic were the individuals who contracted infection or disease. Serological testing demonstrated that the majority of those who had lived at the time of the initial epidemic had pre-existing anti-rubella antibodies.

For a newborn lacking co-functioning acquired/adaptive immunity, its inherent immune response needed to terminate mycobacterium replication is severely taxed. As a consequence, the initial immune response becomes fixed within its immunological memory.

A SPECULATIVE PROPOSAL FOR THE PATHOGENESIS OF CROHNS DISEASE

The way MAP is theorized to be causally related to Crohn's disease differs from the way pathogenic mycobacteria produce disease in humans.

In both Johne's disease in cattle and Crohn's disease, the portal of infection and the target organ of disease are one and the same, namely the gastrointestinal tract. By evolutionary design, the lining and submucosa of the gastrointestinal tract constitute a formidable anatomical and immunological barrier to organism systemic invasion.

The human gastrointestinal tract immune system is a dynamic interplay of checks and balances. Intestinal immune balance is regulated through opposing arms of adaptive immunity.

By their penetration, microbes initiate a pro-inflammatory T-cell response by microorganisms eliciting the development of T-helper-1 (TH1, TH2 or TH17 cells). These pro-inflammatory cells are counterbalanced by the elaboration of regulatory inducible T-cells (Tregs) that have variable expression of Foxhead Box transcription factor (Foxp3f). Treg differentiation results in production of anti-inflammatory cytokines.

In experimental models of colitis, the resultant suppression of TH1 and TH17 cell responses prevent the inflammatory process from developing. The preponderance of MAP therapies that can induce remissions, target effector T-cells or neutralization of selected cytotoxic cytokines underscores the role played by the host immune system in Crohn's disease.

One of the known mechanisms by which mucosal immunity is compromised in the immediate neonatal period involves the relative absence of polysaccharide A (PSA). PSA is produced by symbiotic bacteria within the gastrointestinal microbiota. PSA has been demonstrated to protect the intestines from inflammation by suppressing TH17. Germ free mice have very low numbers of TH17 cells within the lamina propria. The number of TH17 cells corrects to the level observed in control animals with bacterial colonization.

Initially, newborns are not totally dissimilar to germ free animals. PSA is thought to engender mucosal tolerance by promoting the differentiation of functional Treg cells. If an infant is infected when bacterial colonization is incomplete, Foxp3+ Treg cells may not respond appropriately to MAP's antigens. What is theorized is that pathogen challenge when Foxp3+ Treg population is low results in fixation of a pro-inflammatory response.

Tissue studies have demonstrated the fixation of MAP DNA within the lamina propria/mucosa; a requisite for continued antigen processing cells activation.

Individuals with Crohn's disease are thought to lack immune tolerance to subsequent re-exposure to MAP's antigenic array. Whenever MAP or its muramyl dipeptid (MDP) derivatives is processed, pro-inflammatory cytokines that targeting the epithelial sites of antigen attachment, entry and processing are released.

MDP exerts such a powerful polyclonal immune-stimulatory effect on lymphocytes and macrophages that it has been used as a vaccine adjuvant.

The epithelial lining of the gastrointestinal tract possess a remarkable capacity for regeneration. Given the ever increasing presence of viable and non-viable MAP in the food supply, repeated target-specific cytotoxic challenges eventually result in permanent focal destruction in the areas of significant fecal stasis of the lining mucosa of the gastrointestinal tract.

The sustained loss of the epithelial barrier enhances the second element of Crohn's disease: penetration of the submucosa by the previously symbiotic gastrointestinal microbiota. The induced local changes in the oxidation-reduction potential not only allows commensal bacteria to attain disease producing potential, but also alters the composition of the gut bacterial floral.

In Crohn's disease, active MAP replication is theorized not to be a requisite for its induction. What is needed is repetitive re-exposure to MAP's antigen array; hence a proposed mechanism that explains the latency between infection and disease and the reason for the shortening of age of onset for Crohn's disease.

CORRESPONDENCE

E-mail August 12, 2012

Dear Dr. Monif:

"Your suggestion to open a dialogue about collaborative research in MAP dilemma is greatly appreciated. I am not authorized to speak on the behalf of Prof. Pavlik, but I'll inform him and I believe in his positive approach. We are both sure that mycobacteria in the environment and water play an important part in pathogenesis of many chronic inflammatory diseases."

"........ So much data available should beat the buck-passing empty phrase, "Crohn's disease and MAP links still unproven".

Karel Hruska

E-mail August 12, 2012

Dear Drs. Hruska and Pavlik:

"IDI and CGNI are in agreement. We differ only in our approach: i.e. Koch vs. Pasteur."

I have attached the 2012 IDI White Paper (please treat as confidential) and a copy of an open letter that hopefully will be one day published.

IDI concept of the natural history of MAP herbivore infection is different from that advanced in the veterinary literature. Simply, MAP in its spectrum of infection and disease, parallels that documented for Mycobacterium tuberculosis: infection

Gilles R. G. Monif M.D.

is common; disease is significantly rarer. Which occurs is determined by a simple formula:

$$\textbf{Inculum Size } times \textbf{ Virulence}$$
$$divided\ by\ \textbf{Host}$$
$$\textbf{Immunity}.$$

Like tuberculosis, significant compromise of the host's immune system can select for reactivation.

Gilles

E-mail August 17, 2012

Dear Karel and Ivo

Attached are IDI's premises for your review. Right now IDI's first generation solution is to reduce the amount of MAP entering the human food chain through milk. The proposed next generation schema to further reduce the amount even further is vaccination using a novel approach to vaccine development. The problem is that it is too novel……

Gilles

Karel and I differed in our respective approaches to liberating the debate on Crohn's disease from its empty buck-passing phrase of "the link between Crohn's disease and MAP is still unproven". Karel held that distribution of short and provocative premises could influence the discussion necessary to eliminate a hackneyed phrase "links of MAP to Crohn's disease is possible but not confirmed". He firmly believed that science could triumph over politics.

I suffered from a more jaundiced perception of government agencies that tended to function independent of their duties within the public trust.

E-mail September 9, 2012

Dear Karel:

"The MAP dilemma is like trying to eat an elephant. The only way one can "is one bite at a time."

"The comments in the September 2012 Paratuberculosis Newsletter were directed at embarrassing USDA."

"I have great difficulty with the Stabel et al. paper (Appl. Environ. Microbiol. 1997; 63:4975-77)......."

"When the American Academy of Microbiologist indirectly acknowledged the zoonotic character of MAP, FDA convened a panel of PhDs that attempted to defuse the situation. A democratic government is supposed to function in the public trust. Much of the world believes some aspect of that statement."

"When USDA or FDA speaks, their voices are heard afar. I apologize for unloading the soot of my displeasure. I love my country, but fear that it is being transformed into something else."

"Going back to eating an elephant, voluntary programs will not work until there are consequences that bias economic consideration strongly in the favor of doing something. The literature has documented the benefit to producers of putting in place a herd management schema, but to do so still requires

some financial outlay and exposes the producer to some liability. Currently individual producers are hard pressed to make money."

"... The paper on powdered milk is powerful. I strongly concur that milk-related products need to carry some declaration as to the risk assessment of the key ingredients. As you stated milk sold to babies and small children should be designated MAP free..."
"The potential movers are the manufacturers that use milk ..."

Gilles

In September 23, 2012, the Centaur Global Information Network call for mini-reviews on mycobacteria contained the following words:

"A risk, even hypothetical, has to be treated as a risk".

Infectious Diseases Incorporated Premises were published in the CGIN Bulletin' section on Paratuberculosis and Crohn's Disease: Premises and Open Questions. In the December 2012 issue of The Paratuberculosis Newsletter, Soren Nielsen reprinted IDI's premises.

E-mail December 19, 2012

Dear Gilles

Thank you for e-mails on OIE decision. I have been informed few days ago by Ivo (Pavlik) about the video meeting of the IAP officers, who are obviously unable to address Dr. Vallat or to publish arguments against this professional approach of OIE. I really appreciate your precise description. The open discussion on Biomedical Technology, Epidemiology and Food Safety Global Network is ready to publish your opinion with a footnote that the statement of IAP President has been requested and will be published by the same way as soon as it would be available.

The event encourages me in the trust that we should continue in publication of mini-reviews...

Unfortunately, we are nearly totally paralyzed by actions against the five most efficient VRI representatives, suspended by the new management from their positions of deputy director or head of the department without any known reason. Details are not needed, nobody would believe them. It's a cruel life story like an absurd theatre

Please, see the attached draft and let me know if it can be posted and distributed by CGNI.

Karel

Gilles R. G. Monif M.D.

A VOICE WITHIN THE
DOME OF SILENCE

Exerpts from ACVIM Consensus Statement J. Vet. Intern Med. 2012:26:1239-1250

Authors R. W. Sweeney. M.T. Collins, Koets A. P., McGuirk S. M. Roussel A.J.

"...... Some authors argue that there is "no conclusive evidence" that MAP is a cause of Crohn's disease. Direct scientific evidence that MAP is a human pathogen by experimental challenge of young children to fulfill Koch's postulates is unethical. There will never be conclusive evidence. Instead, the scientific community must base any decision on the zoonotic potential of MAP on multiple indirect lines of evidence as discussed below."

"...... Molecular finger-printing demonstrates extensive MAP strain sharing among species. Evidence that MAP can infect taxonomically diverse species is strong."

"........ interestingly, many of the genes associated with a higher frequency of Crohn's disease are also those affecting susceptibility to mycobacterial infections (New Engl. J. Med. 2009; 361:2666-2668)."

"……..Experts suspect that finds humans an abnormal host and adopts a different form, e.g. a spheroclast (cell-deficient) …."

"……..Hill's 10 criteria for causality. For seven of the criteria the authors gauged the evidence as strong or moderate and for two conflicted (Crit. Rev. Microbiol. 2012; 38:52-93)."

Gilles R. G. Monif M.D.

TOO BIG TO TOUCH

E-mail December 18, 2012

Ray Sweeney, Secretary-Treasurer IAP forwards to the general membership the concern of Ramon A. Juste, DVM, PhD, ECSRHM, and President of IAP that the World Organization for Animal Health is working on a new simplified Terrestrial Animal Health Code from which paratuberculosis would be excluded. The reasons advanced are that there is no satisfactory method for detection of infection and the widespread presence of infection represents a hurtle to international trade that would not be justified by the resultant economic losses. He asks the membership to inquire about this issue with their respective national animal health authorities.

The contemplate move by OIE had the potential to open discussion of the MAP dilemma and have different voices heard.

E-mail December 18, 2012

Dear Ray:

"Thank you for the heads up,

To deny that paratuberculosis is a medical as well as veterinary issue that requires an answer/solution and then not to facilitate dissemination of infection and disease on a global level is grossly irresponsible. JDIP needs to flex its intellectual muscle …."

Gilles

E-mail December 20, 2012

To Ramon A. Juste, DVM, PhD, Dip. ECSRHM

Dear Ramon

Because my letter to you is going to be circulated, I needed to make some minor grammatical and content changes.

Please insert this as my response to your e-mail.

Re.: The World Association for Animal Health (OIE)'s proposal to remove paratuberculosis from the Terrestrial Animal

Health Code.

Any decision by the World Organization for Animal Health, OIE, to remove paratuberculosis as a disease entity from the Terrestrial Animal Health Code lacks scientific merit.

If enacted, the consequences will only exacerbate significant agricultural and societal public health issues that, if not addressed, will in time destroy the dairy industry.

To state that there is no satisfactory way to detect animals infected with MAP is a distorted interpretation of the relevant scientific literature. The FUIDI #1 MAP ELISA test specifically addresses the issue of whether detectable MAP is present or not. What has adversely colored the diagnostic literature concerning Mycobacterium avium subspecies paratuberculosis (Map) is the fact that the current commercial MAP ELISA tests certified by the United States Department of Agriculture (USDA) measure anti-MAP antibodies, but the interpretation of a positive test is predicated on the identification of a level of antibody that predicts a high probability of a progression of MAP infection to clinically overt enteritis (Johne's disease) or confirms its presence. A negative commercial MAP ELISA test does not address the issue of whether or not a given animal has ever been infected by MAP.

The decision by USDA to have the MAP ELISA tests represent a statement of probability rather than a valid measurement of the amount of antibody present has permitted infected cows to be transported across state lines and national borders. The net result was not only the introduction of infected animals into uninfected herds, but a dramatic increased prevalence of MAP infection in the national herds. In 2002, 30-40% of U.S. dairy herds had animals with MAP. In 2007, USDA acknowledged that an estimated 70% of U.S. dairy herds contained one or more infected animals (USDA-APHIS Johne's Disease in U.S. Dairies 1991-2007. http://nahms.aphis.usda. gov/ dairy/dairyo7/Dairy 2007-Johnes.pdf.2007). If a test is now used that truly measures the presence or absence of MAP antibodies, the number of infected animals in a large, confined dairy operation may exceed the 2007 seventy percent figure that identified merely one or more MAP infected animals.

Central to the herd monitoring schema proposed by the 2008 National Johne's Disease Control Program for Johne's disease Was the identification and removal of infected animals from the herd. Reducing the introduction of MAP infection and potentially Johne's disease into uninfected herds is largely contingent upon the buyer having the proper information to go along with eyeball analysis of the animal's body condition score.

Quality of merchandise is theoretically addressed through the animal's health certificate. In the United States, revision to parts 71 and 80 of the Code of Federal Regulations (CFR) is supposed to restrict the interstate movement of MAP-infected animals except to recognized slaughter establishments (United States Department of Agriculture Animal Plant Health Inspection Service. 9, Parts 71and 80.2000. Johne's disease in domestic animals: interstate movement. Federal register 65:18875-188879). With an artificially constituted threshold for a positive test, the pertinent CFR regulations do not truly address the quality of merchandise issue. By not stipulating on the animal's certificate of health its MAP status in a manner comparable to Mycobacterium bovis, animals with subclinical disease are and have been transported across state and national boundaries. The decision by USDA not to require a statement as to an animal's MAP status has been a prime factor that undermined its avowed intent to prevent dissemination of MAP into uninfected herds. USDA's decisions have effectively masked the presence of infection in dairy cows, and by so doing exported disease across state and national boundaries.

The Japanese perception that MAP constitutes a potential public health hazard has engendered a different schema (Eiichi M.2012. Epidemiological situation and control strategies for paratuberculosis in Japan. Japanese J. Vet. Res. 60:19s-29s). In accordance with the Act on Domestic Animal Infectious Disease Control, after 1998, every Japanese dairy farm is examined for MAP every five years. Imported cattle are subjected to quarantine in which they are screened using MAP ELISA, fecal culture, analysis of feces for MAP DNA and Johnin skin test. If a new cow is to be introduced into a herd, the recommended procedure is that the cow should be negative in more than two ELISA tests within three-month intervals during the last six months, negative at least once in culture for Map, and kept in quarantine until proven non-infectious. Fifty-four percent of diseased animals detected by the Japanese Animal Quarantine Service came from the United States. Owing to the high antibody threshold for a positive test of the current MAP ELISA tests, the real number of exported infected cows from the United States escaping detection is open to speculation.

The cost of USDA's current policies has been the widespread dissemination of MAP within the nation's dairy and beef herds in the name of protecting agriculture. In trying to placate a threat to the dairy and related industries, USDA has dramatically magnified the threat. Once introduced into the production area, eradication of MAP from that environment is nearly impossible. MAP dissemination within a herd has been documented to be progressive with time.

In its attempt to insulate dairy producers from incurring added production costs embedded in implementing an effective herd management plan, USDA has cost producers money.

Multiple studies have demonstrated a reduction in milk volume and fat content as well as impaired reproductive outcomes occur long before clinical signs become manifested. Instead of having occult losses from a few cows, the producer now had occult losses in milk production, unsuccessful reproductive outcomes, and decreased slaughter weight occurring in the majority of his cows. Once unidentified MAP infection becomes prevalent within a large herd, by itself, small occult milk production losses can become very substantial over time owing to the number of animals now infected.

The more immediate threat to the dairy industry is not whether MAP is the direct (cytokine/tumor necrosis factor) or indirect (induction of an autoimmune response) cause of irritable bowel syndrome and Crohn's disease; it is that milk and milk products may contain an element (the MAP organism) that may be harmful to the public health. A statement to this effect is not on the labels of milk, of baby food made from milk, of products made from milk or powdered milk, etc.

Knowledge supports

1) *MAP is recognized as a zoonotic pathogen;*

2) *the organism has been identified significantly more frequently in disease tissue, milk, and blood from individuals with Crohn's disease than from individuals without gastrointestinal diseases;*

3) *the majority of individuals who consume milk regularly are projected to be infected; and*

4) *even killed MAP release muramyldipeptides that are potent immunomodulators that trigger inflammation.*

To falsify a product label by deleting the inclusion or potential inclusion of a potentially harmful ingredient is inviting civil, if not criminal proceedings.

Recognizing USDA's administrative blunders, the World Organization for Animal Health (OIE) now seeks to whitewash the damage done on a global level using the rationale that because MAP infection is so widespread, continued recognition of MAP as an animal pathogen would only cause economic losses through the restrictions in international animal trade. Ethically, as well as scientifically, OIE has chosen to disregard the preponderance of scientific evidence incriminating MAP in the pathogenesis of human diseases: in particular Crohn's disease and childhood autism.

To do nothing is to do something. The cost of USDA doing nothing has been the widespread dissemination of MAP within the nation's dairy and beef herds in the name of protecting agriculture. OIE is to be congratulated for doing the next best thing to nothing, the wrong thing. Let the International Association for Paratuberculosis (IAP) do the best thing and speak out against a proposal that puts us and our children's children all at a greater risk.

Gilles R. G. Monif, M.D.

E-mail December 20, 2012

Dear Karel:

Battles are ultimately won by the persistent and, if there is a higher power, the righteous. Slowly is good; persistent is best. The key will be to induce the proponents of silence into open discussion. Their weapon has been silence, not science.

What may ultimately bring the zoonotic potential of MAP into open debate is either one of two issues. If anyone had a large human serum bank with corresponding demographic data, it would be demonstrated that a very significant portion of the human population in wealthy industrialized countries have been infected by variants of MAP. (I will either give our MAP technology to an investigator or do the testing per se as a co-investigator.) The second issue is the labeling of food for human consumption. Anything made with milk needs to have on its packaging a statement indicating that the product may contain a zoonotic pathogen, particular baby food made with powdered milk.

When individuals understand that their government has allowed them to be exposed to an organism which is a documented pathogen, the public outrage that has been lacking to date may manifest.

Right now, my science is being compromised by its need to be heard. Until the milk and milk-related industries are assured of their respective survival, they will use every weapon available to them to subvert the issue.

I too am concerned for the number of individuals who will dare to speak out. It is as if we are in a card game in which a 45 automatic triumphs four aces.

What has just been achieved is an energizing of individuals who previously lacked confidence in their beliefs. I like your suggestion to invite individuals to address some limited issue close to their area of expertise that does not put them in harm's way. More focused discussion or data, unless published in open journals, will never see print in veterinary journals for political reasons.

Gilles

****

Before these opinions could be posted and distributed by CGNI, a new management was put in place. Ivo Pavlick left VRI. The five most efficient VRI representatives were suspended from their positions of deputy director or department heads without explanation.

E-mail December 19, 2012

Dear Karel:

I cannot tell you how saddened I am by what is happening. I have held your institute and your country in highest regards for its role in disseminating scientific information.

My mentor, Donald Barron, taught me that the sharing of knowledge is the greatest of all gifts: it enriches both the giver and the receiver.

That IAP officers chose not to put themselves in harm's way is not surprising; yet they can manufacture a response through the 2014 IAP meeting in Parma, Italy..... Between now and then, if Ramon Juste would initiate the dialogue with a strong letter stating his concerns about the pending OIE action, a resultant dialogue could expose the fallacy of OIE's proposal and delineate the projected dire societal consequences.

. . . .

The issue of MAP as a public health hazard is too threatening to those in power. Only when they are assured that their wallets will not be lightened will any progress be made in lessening the consequences of their greed.

Greenstein, Naser, etc. all know the consequences of speaking out. Protect yourself from evil. The American Indians recognized the negative force that emanates from gold and shun it.

Gilles

E-mail December 21, 2012

The president of IAP asked that the content of his e-mail of December 21, 2012 not be published.

The official position of the Spanish government is to be one of concurrence with any decision of OIE.

E-mail January 2, 2013

Dear Gilles and Ivo,

Few comments received from Prof. George Poppensiek, USA, Prof. Kouba, Former Chief, Animal Health Service, FAO, Joe Falkinham, A. Maraz, Hungary.

Seven new subscribers for CGNI 08 Mycobacterial diseases from USA, Egypt, Pakistan, Malaysia.

Karel

In 2014, Professor Karel Hruska "retired" from VRI.

PREVENTION OF CROHN'S DISEASE

Milk and milk-derived products are backed by powerful economic interests that are too big to .... (The 20th century's catch phrase for "protected at the public's expense"). Without their consent, a resolution, more probably than not, can't be achieved.

Crohn's disease is costing the United States government billions of taxpayer's dollars annually. Too many individuals are being forced out of the work force in their prime earning years. Others have to seek lesser employment to accommodate their disease.

The cost of achieving a remission using TNF "knock out" drugs is now a big ticket item for individuals, insurance companies, and governments. On an annual basis, the increasing number of citizens becoming afflicted with Crohn's will eventually force governments to choose among their funding priorities.

Contrary to existing laws validated by the United States Supreme Court, little to nothing will be agreed to by those who control USDA and FDA until accommodations are in place that will economically protect agribusiness.

The Federal Meat Inspection Act (21 U.S.C.601 et seq.), the Poultry Product Inspection Act, (21m U.S.C. 451 et seq.) and the Federal Food, Drug, and Cosmetic Act (21 U.S.C.321 et seq.) identify a food as being "adulterated" if it bears or contains any "poisonous or deleterious substance" which may render it injurious to health and is not neutralized by its subsequent processing. Products that are adulterated under these laws cannot enter into commerce for food consumption.

The Federal Meat Act's provision number five defines adulterated as being "If it contains any added poisonous or other added deleterious ingredient which may render such article injurious to health."

In 2011, then Senator Kristen Gillibrand attempted to introduce a bill to widen the definition of adulterated food products and add criminal penalties for food manufacturers that knowingly introduced contaminated food into commerce. Specifically, Gillibrand's bill sought to amend the Federal Meat Inspection Act so that the term "adulterated" included emerging pathogens "associated with actual or potential human illness or death." FDA, which is charged with regulating and enforcing laws on food safety, is said to have advocated against its adoption.

Both USDA and FDA have had evidence-based substantiation, not just that MAP was intimately meshed with Crohn's disease, but more specifically, that MAP in milk, infant formula, yogurt and soft cheeses constituted a hypothetical risk to the public health. Despite possessing on-going knowledge of the proposed relationship, FDA has allowed third parties to use the government's implied guarantee of food safety without providing appropriate information that would have allowed an individual of average intelligence to make an informed choice.

In defiance of the Rio Declaration on Food Safety, the Sanitary and Phytosanitary Measures of the World Trade Organization and the United States Congress, USDA and FDA have allegedly taken it upon themselves to implement a course of action that has put individuals potentially in harm's way.

For FDA *"Where there are threats of serious or irreversible damage, lack of full knowledge shall not be used as reasoning for postponing cost-effective measures ...."* has little apparent significance.

Unless the Rio Declaration is but an exercise in penmanship, the U.S. government pledged itself to treat a hypothetical risk as a risk. A hypothetical risk to the public health, particularly one substantiated by scientific proofs, must be treated as a risk. To act a government, doesn't have to believe that MAP is the cause of Crohn's disease. It has only to accept that a hypothetical risk to the public health is present.

The cost-effective measures that FDA refused to implement are and were extraordinarily simple: **make certain that the milk processed for infant formula or milk used in the first four weeks of life is MAP free.** Only bulk tank milk certified as being MAP free should be used for inclusion in infant formula and milk sold in stores specifically marked for infant feeding during the first four weeks of age.

The most cost effective way for FDA and USDA to protect agribusiness' business stake in the nation's economy will be to utilize federal funds to, using the strongest possible language, inform women of the wisdom of breast feeding their newborns through the age of four weeks.

Based upon the implied postulate deductable from epidemiological data, USDA and FDA can subsequently reassure the world that they could continue to enjoy consumption of milk, ice cream, cheeses and yogurt with possibly little fear of adverse consequences.

To have acted in a preventive manner, all that was required was for USDA and FDA to acknowledge that MAP in milk and milk-based products constitutes "a hypothetical risk" to the public welfare.

In the longer run, more probably than not, governments need to reduce the amount of MAP entering the food supply. One component in the equation that selects for infection or disease is the size of the inoculum. For Crohn's disease, size of the inoculum translates into the magnitude of the initial antigenic challenge.

The implied third party manipulation of the public health and the resultant betrayal of the public trust by government agencies are not matters that should be treated lightly, less inaction unmask the lack of an underlying democratic process.

Negligent Entrustment is a cause of action in tort law that arises where one party (the entrustor) is held for negligence because the party negligently provided another party (the trustee) with a dangerous instrument, and the entrusted party caused injury to a third party with that instrument.

FDA has been able to justify its inaction by reference to its internally engendered guidelines that require that proof be conclusive before labeling a substance a hazard or potential hazard to the public health. Having made conclusiveness the requirement for any form of action, FDA has made it near certain that the cause of Crohn's disease could never be successfully argued within the federal court system without costly retribution by industry.

Being conversant with the literature and possessing in depth knowledge of the epidemiological data and diagnostic methodology, USDA and FDA appear to have crossed the fine line separating negligent entrustment from criminal negligence.

Criminal Negligence arises when an accused has not actually foreseen the potentially adverse consequences to the planned actions, and has gone ahead, exposing a particular individual or unknown victim to the risk of suffering injury or loss. It can be argued that USDA and FDA have endangered the safety of others in circumstances where, given the same information, a reasonable person armed with the same knowledge would have foreseen the injury and taken preventive measures.

Crohn's disease has been directly and indirectly responsible for the premature death of thousands of U.S, citizens. Once the hypothesis of causality had been advanced and reasonably substantiated, the response of an individual of average intelligence was stated in Lord Justice Phillips' report to Her Majesty's Government and the United Kingdom Food Standard Agency Report.

Between 2002 and 2015, an estimated 400,000 new cases of Crohn's disease have occurred. Those responsible for alleged breaches of fiduciary responsibility will eventually retire with pensions paid for by the very people they have placed in harm's way.

The public trust is an area of law for which governments are the trustees. Ethically and legally, public trust rights are just that, rights. Citizens within a democracy have the enduring right to the resources upon which their well-being and very survival depend. In supporting agendas that serve corporative interests, have not selected government agencies become complicit in the death of U.S. citizens?

"To do nothing is to do something." The cost of USDA sitting on its hands has been the widespread dissemination of MAP within the nation's dairy herds. The next cost of doing nothing, more likely than not, has been the placing of probably hundreds of thousands if not multiple millions of Americans, without their knowledge or consent, potentially in harm's way. Even more damning is endangering of the welfare of future generations.

But by far the greatest cost of doing nothing is damaging the belief that the United States is a country for the people.

APPENDIX

EPILOGUE

If the Hruska postulate can't be discredited, hundreds of thousands of individuals afflicted with a life-changing disease are a terrible price to pay in the service of agribusiness. Billions of dollars are spent annually to apply pharmaceutical Band-Aids to abate symptoms and to prevent possible death from Crohn's disease complications.

Why is Crohn's disease a new disease entity in the twentieth century?

The epidemic increase in the number of Crohn's disease cases, particularly during the past three decades, imposes a more imposing **Why?**

The proposed explanation as to the **Why?s** has an answer in the layering of conforming scientific observation.

The book is a scientific discussion as to the pathogenesis of Crohn's disease. The right to express a scientific opinion is protected by the First and Fourth Amendment rights of the United States Constitution. A reference list worthy of being read has been supplied for those who wish to argue against the measures that can be taken to prevent Crohn's disease.

Given what has happened to other investigators whose findings implicate a relationship between MAP and Crohn's disease, it is anticipated that a horde of the Controllers' lawyers will descend and attempt to financially punish those who still chose not to sin by silence.

If the Controllers really want to protect a collective agribusiness bottom line, they have merely to instruct USDA to fund a campaign that aggressively advocates breast feeding of all babies through the first few weeks of life and then, have USDA set "comfortable" limits on the amount of MAP allowable in bulk tank milk.

As to hypothetical loss of agribusiness revenue due to the discussion of the consequences of USDA's mismanagement of the MAP issue, the Controllers should arrange for USDA to have them reimbursed for any theoretical losses from the public treasury.

The intimidating threat of consequences has caused most investigators involved with the MAP dilemma to sin by silence rather than pursue their scientific convictions. The cost of speaking out has been career ruining for those who dared to speak out. This fact magnifies the courage demonstrated by Karel Hruska and Ivo Pavlik. As soldiers with a pen, they have paid dearly for having pursued a scientific truth in the service of the us all.

Science will ultimately thank Karel Hruska for delineating a mechanism by which a so-called "auto-immune diseases" can be initiated. The mechanism described has the potential to unchain other disease entities from the thought- paralyzing diagnosis of being "auto-immune diseases".

REFERENCES

Agriculture (USDA). (2000). United States Food Safety System Country Report. Annex II: Precaution in US food safety decision making. Washington, DC: US FDA/USDA. Available on the World Wide Web: http://www.foodsafety.gov/~fsg/fssyst4.html.

Allen A. J., Parks K. T., Barrington G. M., Lahmers K.K., Abdellrazeq G. S., Rihan H. M., Sreevatsan S., Davies C., Hamilton M. J., Davis W. C.: Experimental infection of a bovine model with human isolates of *Mycobacterium avium* subspecies *paratuberculosis*. Vet. Immun. Immunopath. 2011; 141:258-266

Autschbach F., Eisold S., Hinz U., Zinser S., Linnebacher M., Giese T., Löffler T., Büchler, M.W., Schmidt J.: High prevalence of *Mycobacterium avium* subspecies *paratuberculosis* IS900 DNA in gut tissue from individuals with Crohn's disease. Gut 2005; 54:944-949

Ayele W.Y., Svastova P, Roubal P., Bartos M, Pavlik I.: *Mycobacterium avium* subspecies *paratuberculosis* cultured from locally and commercially pasteurized cow's milk in the Czech Republic. Appl. Envir. Microbiol. 2005; 71:1210-1214

Bailey M. Haverson K.: The postnatal development of the mucosal immune system and mucosal tolerance in domestic animals. Vet. Res. 2006; 7: 443-453

Barclay A.R., Russell R. K., Wilson M. L., Gilmour W. H., Satsangi J., Wilson D.C.: Systemic review: The role of breastfeeding in the development of pediatric inflammatory bowel disease. J. Pediat. 2009; 155:421-426

Belkaid Y., Tarbell K.: regulatory T-cells in control of host-microorganism interactions. Annu. Rev. Immunol 2009; 226:219-233

Bergstrand O., Hellers G.: Breastfeeding during infancy in patients who later develop Crohn's disease. Scand. J. Gastroenterol. 1983; 18:903-906

Buergelt C. D., Williams J. E., Monif G. R. G.: Spontaneous clinical remission of Johne's disease in a Holstein cow, Int. J. Applied Res. Vet. Med. 2004; 2:126-128,

Buergelt C. D. Williams J. E., Decker J. H., Monif G., Pinedo P.: Nested polymerase chain reaction for detection of *Mycobacterium avium* subspecies *paratuberculosis* in bovine allantoic fluid and fetuses. Proceedings of 9th ICP 2007: 91-93

Buergelt, C. D. Williams J. E. Monif G. R. G.: *In utero* infection of pregnant cattle by *Mycobacterium avium* subspecies *paratuberculosis* detected by nested polymerase chain reaction. Intn. J. Appl. Res. Vet. Med. 2003; 1:279-284

Bull T.J, McMinn E.J., Sidi-Boumedine K., Skull, A., Durkin D., Neild P., Rhodes G., Pickup R., Hermon-Taylor J.: Detection and verification of *Mycobacterium avium* subspecies *paratuberculosis* in fresh ileocolonic mucosal biopsy from individuals with and without Crohn's disease. J. Clin. Microbiol. 2003; 41:2915-2923

Byun, E.H., Kim, W.S., Kim, J.S., Won, C. J., Choi, H. G., Kim, H.J., Cho, S. N., Lee, K., Zhang, T., Hur, G.M., ShIn, S.J. *Mycobacterium* paratuberculosis CobT activates dendritic cells via engagement of toll-like receptor 4 resulting in Th1 cell expansion. Journal of Biological Chemistry 2012: 287:38609-38624

Clark D. L. Jr., Anderson J. L., Kozickowski J. J., Ellingson J. L. E.: Detection of *Mycobacterium avium* subspecies *paratuberculosis* in cheese curds purchased in Wisconsin and Minnesota. Molecular Cell. Probes 2006; 20:197-202

Chiodini R.J.: Crohn's disease and the mycobacterioses: a review and comparison of two entities, Clin. Microbiol. Rev. 1989; 2:90-117

Chiodini R.J, Rossiter C. A: Paratuberculosis: a potential zoonosis. Vet. Clin. North Am.: Food Animal Practices. 1996; 12:457-467

Collin M.T.: Summation. 9th ICP, Tsukuba, Japan.2007": pp. 354-355

Coombes J. L., Robinson N. J., Maloy K. J., Uhlig H. H., Powrie F., regulatory T cells and intestinal homeostasis. Immunol. Rev. 2005; 204:184-194

Cousins D. V. Whittington R. Marsh I, Masters R., Evans R.J., Kluver P.: Mycobacteria distinct from *Mycobacterium avium* subspecies *paratuberculosis* isolated from faeces of ruminants possess IS900-like sequences detectable by polymerase chain reaction: implication for diagnosis. Mol. Cell Probes 1999; 14:431-442

Crohn's Disease 2000: p6. National Association for Colitis and Crohn's Disease (NACC) www.nacc.org.uk

Deng W. Y., Xie J. P.:NOD2 signaling and role in pathogenic mycobacterium recognition, infection, and immunity. Cell. Physiol. Biochem. 2012; 30:953-963

Dong C.: Diversification of T-helper lineage. Finding the family root of TH17-producing cells. Nat. Rev. Immunol. 2006; 6:329-333

Ellingson J.L., Anderson J.L., Koziczkowski J.J., Radcliff R.P., Sloan S.J., Allen S.E., Sullivan N.M.: Detection of viable *Mycobacterium avium* subspecies *paratuberculosis* in retail pasteurized whole milk by two culture methods and PCR. J. Food Prot. 2005: 68:966-972

Eisenberg S. W., Nielsen M., Santema W. Houwers D. L., Heederik D., Koets A. P.: Detection of spatial and temporal spread of *Mycobacterium avium* subsp. *paratuberculosis* in the environment of a cattle farm through bio-aerosols. Vet. Microbiol. 2010; 143:284-292

Englund S., Bolske G, Johansson K. E.: An IS900-like sequence found in a Mycobacterium sp. other than *Mycobacterium avium* subspecies *paratuberculosis*. FEMS Microbiol. Lett. 2002; 209:267-271

European Commission Report of the Scientific Committee on Animal Health and Animal Welfare: Possible links between Crohn's disease and paratuberculosis, 2000; pp1-76

Feuerer M, Hill J. A., Mathis D., Benoist C.: Foxp3+ regulatory T cells: Differentiation, specification, subphenotypes. Nat. Immunol. 2009; 10:689-695

Frothingham C. R.: Evolutionary bottlenecks in the agents of tuberculosis, leprosy and paratuberculosis. Med. Hypothesis 1999; 52: 95-99

Ghadiali A. H., Strother M., Naser S. A. et al.: *Mycobacterium avium* subsp. *paratuberculosis* strains isolated from Crohn's disease patients and animal species exhibit similar polymorphic locus patterns. J. Clin. Microbiol. 2004; 42:5345-5348.

Giese S.B., Ahrens P.: Detection of *Mycobacterium avium* subsp. *paratuberculosis* in milk from clinically affected cows by PCR and culture. Vet. Microbiol. 2000; 77:291-297

Grant I. R., Ball H. J., Neill S. D., Rowe M. T.: Inactivation of *Mycobacterium paratuberculosis* in cow's milk at pasteurization temperatures. Appl. Environ. Microbiol. 1996; 62:631-636

Grant I. R., Ball H. J., Condron R. J.: Effect of high-temperature short-time HTST pasteurization on milk containing low levels of *Mycobacterium paratuberculosis*. Ltt. Appl. Microbiol. 1998; 26:166-170

Grant I. R., Ball H. J., Rowe M. T.: Incidence of *Mycobacterium paratuberculosis* in bulk raw and commercially pasteurized milk from approved dairy processing establishments in the United Kingdom. Appl. Envir. Microbiol. 2002; 68:2428-2435

Harris N. B., Barleta R. G.: *Mycobacterium avium* subspecies *paratuberculosis* in veterinary medicine. Clin. Microbiol. Rev. 2001; 14:489-503

Herman-Taylor J., Barnes N., Clarke C., Finlayson C.: Grand round – *Mycobacterium paratuberculosis cervical* lymphadenitis, followed five years later by terminal ileitis similar to Crohn's disease. Brit. Med. J. 1998; 316:449-453

Hermon-Taylor J., Bull T. J., Sheridan J. M., Cheng J., Stellakis M. L., Sumar N.: Causation of Crohn's disease by *Mycobacterium avium* subspecies *paratuberculosis.* Canadian J. Gastroenerol. 2000, 14:521-523

Hermon-Taylor J.: *Mycobacterium avium* subspecies *paratuberculosis:*in the causation of Crohn's disease World J. Gastroenterrol. 2000; 6:630-632

Hermon-Taylor J.: Protagonist: *Mycobacterium avium* subspecies *paratuberculosis is acause of Crohn's disease. Gut 2001; 49:755-5*

Hermon-Taylor J.:. Mycobacterium avium subspecies paratuberculosis, Crohn's disease and the doomsday scenario. Gut Pathogens 2009; 1:15-20

Hornell A., Lagstrom H., Lande B., Thorsdottri I.: Breastfeeding, introduction of other foods effect on health a systematic literature review for the 5th Nordic Nutrition Recommendations. Food Nut Res.2013, 57

Horta B., Bahl R., Martinez J, Victora C.: Evidence on the long term effects of breast feeding: systemic reviews and meta-analysis: World Health Organization: http:// wholibdoc.who.int/publications/2007/9789241

Hruska K., Bartos M., Kralik P., Pavlik I.: *Mycobacterium avium* subspecies *paratuberculosis* in powdered infant milk: paratuberculosis in cattle – the public health problem to be solved. Veterinarni Medicina 2005; 327-335 http://vri.cs/docs/vetmed/50-8-327.pdf

Hruska K., Slama J., Kralik P., Pavlik I. *Mycobacterium avium* subsp. *paratuberculosis* in powdered milk: F57 competitive real time PCR: Veterinarni Medicina 2011; 226-230 http://vri.cs/docs/vetmed/56-5-226.pdf

Hruska K., Pavlik: Crohn's disease and related inflammatory diseases: from a single hypothesis to one "superhypothesis." Veterinarni Medicina 2014; 59-583-630 http://vri.cs/docs/vetmed/59-12-583.pdf

http://www.crohns.org/congress/index.htm

http://vri.cz/docs/vetmed/59-12-583.pdf

Ikonomoplus J., Pavlik I., Bartos M., Svastova P., Ayele W. Y., Roubal P., Lukas J., Cook N., Gazouli M.: Detection of *Mycobacterium avium* subspecies *paratuberculosis* in retail cheese from Greece and Czech Republic. Appl. Environ. Microbiol. 2005; 71:8935-9036

Ip S., Chung M., Raman G., Chew P. et al.: Breastfeeding and maternal and infant health outcomes in developed countries, Evid. Rep. Technol. Assess. 2007; 153:1-186 http://www.ncbi.nlm.nih.gov/

Juste R. A., Elguezabal N., Pavon A., Garrido J. M., Geijo M., Sevilla I, Cabriada J.L., Tejada A., Garcia-Campos F., Casado R. Ochontorena I., Izeta A.: Association between *Mycobacterium avium* subsp. *paratuberculosis* DNA in blood and cellular and humeral immune response in inflammatory bowel disease patents and controls. Intern J. Infect. Dis. 2009;13:247-254 27.

Karina C., Huberman Y. D., Paolicchi; Viability of *Mycobacterium avium* subsp. paratuberculosis during traditional elaboration and storage of yogurt, Proceedings of the 10th ICP 2009: p.277

Kennedy D., Benedictus G.: It's time for IAP to take the lead on international spread of paratuberculosis. Paratb. Newsletter December 2014: pp. 52-53

Kirkwood CD, Wagner J, Boniface K, Vaughan J, Michalski WP, Catto-Smith AG, Cameron DJ, Bishop RF: *Mycobacterium avium* subspecies *paratuberculosis* in children with early-onset Crohn's disease. *Inflamm Bowel Dis* 2009; 15:1643-55

Klement E., Cohen R. V., Boxman J. Joseph A., Reif S.: Breastfeeding and risk of inflammatory bowel disease: a systemic review with meta-analysis. Am J. Clin. Nutr. 2004; 80:1342-1352

Maynard C.L., Weaver C. T.: Diversity in the contribution of interlukin-10 to T cell-mediated immune regulation. Immunol. Rev. 2008; 226:219-233

Mazmanian S. K., Round J. L., Kasper D. L.: A microbial symbiosis factor prevents intestinal inflammatory disease. Nature 2008; 453:620-625

Mazmanian S. K., Round J. L., Kasper D.L.: A microbial symbiosis factor prevents intestinal inflammatory disease. Immunol Rev. 2008; 453;620-625

Mendoza J. L, San-Pedro A., Culebras E., Cies R., Taxonera C., Lana R., Urcelay E., de la Torre F., Picazo J.J., Diaz Rubio M.: High prevalence of viable *Mycobacterium avium* subspecies *paratuberculosis* in Crohn's disease. World J. Gastroenterology 2010; 16:4558-4563

Millar D., Ford J., Sanderson J., Withey S., Tizard M., Doran T., Hermon-Taylor J.: IS 900 PCR to detect *Mycobacterium avium* subspecies *paratuberculosis* in retail supplies of whole pasteurized milk in England and Wales. Appl. Environ. Microbiol. 1996; 62:3454

Monif G. R. G. Viral Infections of the Human Fetus. New York, Macmillan 1969

Monif G. R. G.: Certification of Health for Dairy Cows. Paratb. Newsletter. December 2008: pp. 13-14

Monif G. R. G.: What if? A contrarian's questioning of the natural history of bovine infection due to *Mycobacterium avium* subspecies *paratuberculosis* Paratb. Newsletter June 2008: pp. 10-11

Monif G. R. G. Williams J. E. Sheppard B. J.: Equine Johne's disease: Are equine *Mycobacterium avium* and *M. avium* subsp. *paratuberculosis* truly *M. avium* and *M. avium* subspecies *paratuberculosis.* Paratb. Newsletter September 2008: p.13

Monif G. R. G.: The difference between an A and a THE. Paratb. Newsletter March 2009: pp. 6-7

Monif G. R. G.: An ounce of prevention is worth more than a pound of cure: Certificates of animal health must be just that. Paratb. Newsletter. December 2009: pp. 40-41

Monif G. R. G., Williams J.E.: The natural history of *Mycobacterium avium* subspecies *paratuberculosis* as interpreted by the FUIDI #2 MAP test. Proceedings of 10th ICP. 2009; p. 164, Minneapolis, MN

Monif G. R. G., Lin, T.L. Williams J. E. Wu C. C.: Significance of heavy fecal shedding of *Mycobacterium avium* subspecies *paratuberculosis* (MAP): Comparison of fecal culture, real-time and nested PCR testing. Proceedings of 10th ICP 2009: pp.41-43. Minneapolis, MN

Monif, G. R. G. The FUIDI Herd Management Schema: Proceedings of 10th ICP 2009: pp. 204-206. Minneapolis, MN

Monif G. R. G., Williams J.E.: Significance of double MAP agar gel immunodiffusion precipitation bands. Proceedings of 10th ICP 2009: pp. 38-40. Minneapolis, MN

Monif, G. R. G., Lin T. L., Williams, J. E., Wu C.C.: The prevalence of possible *Mycobacterium avium* subspecies *avium* in fecal samples of dairy cows. Proceedings of 10th ICP 2009: pp.165-167. Minneapolis, MN

Monif G. R. G.: Two worlds on a collision course. Proceedings of 10th ICP 2009: pp. 278-280. Minneapolis, MN

Monif G. R. G.: Testing bovine milk for the presence of antibodies to *Mycobacterium avium* subspecies *paratuberculosis*. Paratb. Newsletter June 2009: p.16

Monif G. R. G.: Turmoil in U.S. dairy industry: An opportunity to improve herd quality with respect to *Mycobacterium avium* subspecies *paratuberculosis*. Paratb. Newsletter September 2009: pp.32-33

Monif, G. R. G.: Insanity. Paratb. Newsletter December 2010: pp. 97- 09

Monif G. R. G.: Cytomegaloviruses. In Infectious Diseases in Obstetrics and Gynecology. Sixth edition. Editors Gilles R. G. Monif and David A. Baker 2010 Informa, London, United Kingdom

Monif G. R. G.: Enteroviruses. In Infectious Diseases in Obstetrics and Gynecology. Sixth edition. Editors Gilles R. G. Monif and David A. Baker 2010 Informa, London, United Kingdom

Monif, G.R.G: Infectious Diseases Incorporated FUIDI Premises. CNG Information 2012-08-21-132, http:// centaur.vri.cz/docs/ Reports2012/FUIDI_premises CGNI_ 120818E_Reports.pdf

Monif G. R. G., Williams J. E.: The significance of a negative MAP ELISA test for *Mycobacterium avium* subspecies *paratuberculosis,* Int. J. Appl. Res. Vet. Med. 2012; 11:116-122

Monif G. R. G.: The MAP milk tax. Paratb. Newsletter June 2014: pp. 19-22 Monif G. R. G. Williams J.E.: Relationship of intestinal eosinophilia and acid-fast bacilli in Johne's disease. Intern J. Appl. Res. Vet. Med. 2015; 13:147-149

Momotani E; http://www.springerplus.com/content/pdf/21 93-1801-1-47.pdf

Monotami.: Epidemiological situation and control strategies for paratuberculosis in Japan. Japanese J. Vet. Res. 2012; 60:19s-29s

Mowat A. M.: Dendritic cells and immune responses to orally administered antigens. Vaccines. 2005; 23:1797-99

Nacy C., Buckley M.: *Mycobacterium avium paratuberculosis*: Infrequent Human Pathogen or Public Health threat?

Report from the American Academy of Microbiology 2008. p. 1-37.

Naser S.A., Schwartz D., Shafran I.: Isolation of *Mycobacterium avium* subspecies *paratuberculosis* (MAP) from breast milk of patients with Crohn's disease. Am. J. Gastroenterol. 2000; 95:1094-1095

Naser S.A., Ghobrial G., Romero C., Valentine J. F.: Culture of *Mycobacterium avium* subspecies *paratuberculosis* (MAP) from the blood of patients with Crohn's disease. Lancet 2004; 364:1039-1044

Naser S. A., Collins M. T., Crawford J. T., Valentine J. F.: Culture of *Mycobacterium avium* subspecies *paratuberculosis* (MAP) from the blood of patients with Crohn's disease: A follow-up blind multicenter investigation. *The Open Inflam. J.* 2009; 2:22-23

Niess J.H., Leithauser F., Alder G., Reimann J.: Commensal gut flora drives the expansion of pro-inflammatory CD4 T cells in the colonic lamina propria under normal and inflammatory conditions. J. Immunol. 2008; 180:559-568

Olbe L. Concept of Crohn's disease being conditioned by four main component and irritable bowel disease being an incomplete Crohn's disease. Scand. J. Gastroenterol. 2008 43:234-241

Paolicchi, F., Cirone, K., Morsella, C., Gioffre, A. (2012). First isolation of Mycobacterium avium subspecies paratuberculosis from commercial pasteurized milk in

Argentina. Brazilian Journal of Microbiology. 2012: 43: 1034-1037

Pinedo P. J., Williams J. E., Monif G. R. G., Rae D. O., Buergelt C. D.: *Mycobacterium* paratuberculosis shedding into milk: association of ELISA seroreactivity with DNA detection in milk. Int. J. Appl. Res. Vet. Med.2008; 6:137-144

Round J. L., Mazmanian S. Inducible Foxp3+ regulatory T-cell development by a commensal bacterium of the intestinal tract. Proc. Natl. Acad. Sci. 2010; 107:12204-12309

Rubery E.: A review of the evidence for a link between *Mycobacterium avium* subspecies *paratuberculosis* (MAP) and Crohn's disease (CD) in humans. A Report for the Food Standard Agency, June 2001.

Saxegaard F., Baess I. Relationship between *Mycobacterium avium, Mycobacterium paratuberculosis* and "wood pigeom mycobacterium. Acta Path. Microbiol. Immunol. Scand. 1988: 96:37-42

Scana A. M., Bull T. J., Cannas S., Sanderson J. D., Sechi L. A., Dettori G., Zanetti S., Hermon-Taylor J.: *Mycobacteriumm avium* subspecies *paratuberculosis* infection of irritable bowel syndrome and comparison with Crohn's disease and Johne's disease: common neural and immune pathogenicities. J. Clin. Microbiol 2007; 45:3883-890

Schleig P.M., Buergelt C. D. Davis J. K., Williams E., Monif G. R. G. Davidson M. K.: Attachment of *Mycobacterium avium* subspecies *paratuberculosis* to bovine intestinal organ cultures; method development and strain differences. Vet. Microbio.l 2005; 108:271-279

Schwartz A.: National Johne's Disease Control Program Strategic Plan. USDA October 23, 2008

Sechi L. A., Scanu A. M., Molicotti P., Molicotti P., Cannes S., Mura M., Dettori G., Fadda G., Zanetti S.: Detection and isolation of *Mycobacterium avium* subspecies *paratuberculosis* from intestinal biopsies of patients with and without Crohn's disease in Sardinia. Am. J. Gastroenteriol. 2005; 100:1529-1534

Secretariat of the Convention on Biological Diversity (SCBD). (2000). *Cartagena protocol on biosafety to the convention on biological diversity: Text and annexes*. Montreal: SCBD.

Strobert W. Vitamin A rewrite the ABC of oral immunity. Mucosal Immun. 2008:92-95

Sheppard B. J., Hawkins I, Williams. E., Monif G. R. G.: Equine granulomatous enteritis due to *Mycobacterium avium* subsp. *paratuberculosis*. Paratb. Newsletter March 2008: p. 9

Sockett D. C.: Johne's disease eradication and control: regulation implications. Vet. Clin. North Am. Food Anim. Practice 1996; 12:431-440

Stabel J. R., Steadham E, M., Bolin C. A.: Heat inactivation of *Mycobacterium paratuberculosis* in raw milk: are current pasteurization conditions effective/ Appl. Environ. Microbiol. 1997; 63:4975-48977

Such L, A.., Scan A. M., Manicotti P., Cannes S. et al.: detection and isolation of *Mycobacterium avium* subspecies *paratuberculosis* from intestinal biopsies of patients with and without Crohn's disease in Sardinia. Am. J. Gastroenterol. 2005; 100:1529-1523

Timms, V. J., Gehringer, M. M., Mitchell, H. M., Daskalopoulos, G., Neilan, B.A. (2011). How accurately can we detect Mycobacterium avium subsp paratuberculosis infection? Journal of Microbiological Methods. 2011; 85:1-8

Thayer Jr W.R., Coutu J.A., Chiodini R.J., Van Kruiningen H. J., Merkal R. S. Possible role of mycobacteria in inflammatory bowel disease. II. Mycobacterial antibodies in Crohn's disease. *Dig Dis Sci* 1984; 29:1080-1085

Turenne C. Y., Wallace R. Jr., Behr M. A.: Mycobacterium avium in the postgenomic era, Clin. Microbiol. Rev. 2007; 20: 205-229

Uniform program standards for the voluntary Johne's disease control program. United States Department of Agriculture, Animal and Plant Health Inspection Service. APIS 91-45-014)

United Nations Environment Programme (UNEP). (1992). Rio declaration on environment and development. Made at the *United Nations Conference on Environment and Development*, Rio de Janeiro, Brazil. Available on the World

Wide Web: http: //www.unep.org/ Documents/Default. asp?DocumentID=78&ArticleID-1163.

United States Food and Drug Administration (US FDA). (1996). Food labeling: Health claims and label statements; Folate and neural tube defects. Proposed rule. *Federal Register*, 61, 8750-8781.

United States Food and Drug Administration (US FDA) and the United States Department of Agriculture (USDA). (2000). United States Food Safety System Country Report. Annex II: Precaution in US food safety decision making. Washington, DC: US FDA/USDA. Available on the World Wide Web: http://www.foodsafety.gov/~fsg/fssyst4.html

United States Department of Agriculture Animal Plant Health Inspection Service. 9, Parts 71 and 80.2000. Johne's disease in domestic animals: interstate movement. Federal register 65:18875-18879

USDA-APHIS Johne's Disease in U.S. Dairies 1991-2007. http:// nahms.aphis.usda.gov/dairy/dairyo7/Dairy 2007-Jo hnes.pdf

Van Brandt, L., Coudijzer, K., Herman, L., Michiels, C., Hendrickx, M., Vlaemynck, G. (2011). Survival of Mycobacterium avium ssp paratuberculosis in yoghurt and in commercial fermented milk products containing probiotic cultures. Journal of Applied Microbiology. 2011; 110:1252-1261

Van Kruiningen H.J. Lack of support for a common etiology in Johne's disease of animals and Crohn's disease in humans. *Inflamm Bowel Dis* 1999; 5:183-91

Van Kruiningen H. J., Ruiz B., Gumprecht L. Experimental disease in young chickens induced by a *Mycobacterium paratuberculosis* isolate from a patient with Crohn's disease. *Can J Vet Res* 1991; 55:199-202

Van Kruiningen H. J.: Where are weapons of mass destruction - *Mycobacterium paratuberculosis* in Crohn's disease? J. Crohn's Colitis 2011; 5:6338-6441

Williams E., Monif G. R. G., Buergelt C. D.: Comparative analysis of different MAP ELISA test. Paratb. Newsletter March 2008: p.9

Williams E., Monif G. R. G.: Comparative MAP ELISA tests done with necropsy documented Johne's disease. Paratb. Newsletter, March 2008: pp.9-10

Williams E., Monif G. R. G.: Impact of Immunonutritional dietary additives on AGID positive cows with Johne's disease. Paratb. Newsletter March 2008 pp.7-8

Williams E., Monif G. R. G.: Persistent bovine fecal shedding in the first month. Paratb. Newletter June 2008: p. 9

William J. E., Steinfieldt K., Monif G. R. G.: Duration of maternally acquired antibodies to *Mycobacterium avium* subsp. *paratuberculosis.* Paratb. Newsletter June 2008: p 10

Williams J.E., Buergelt C. D., Pinedo P., Monif G. R. G.: Use of blotted tissue impressions for rapid PCR identification of *Mycobacterium avium* subsp. *paratuberculosis*. Paratb. Newsletter September 2008: pp.10-12

Williams J. E., Monif G. R. G.: A procedure to assist in the identification of slow growing mycobacterium from slants. Paratb Newsletter March 2009: p. 5

Williams J. E., Pinedo P. J., Monif G. R. G.: Comparative IS900 and IS1311 direct fecal Mycobacterium avium subspecies paratuberculosis nested PCR tests: Significance of Disparities, Proceedings of 10th ICP 2009 44-46

Wisziewska-Laszczych Szteyn L., Smolinska A.: Analysis of correlation between the correlation of anti-MAP antibodies in blood serum and presence of DNA-MAP in milk. Polish J. Vet Sci. 2009; 23:379-383

World Trade Organization (WTO). (1994). The WTO Agreement on the Application of Sanitary and Phytosanitary Measures (SPS Agreement). Web: http://www.wto.org/tratop_e/sps_e/spsagr_e.htm

Wu C. C., Lin T. L., Monif G.R. G.: Comparison of direct fetal culture and direct fecal real-time PCR in the identification of *Mycobacterium avium subsp. paratuberculosis* in fecal specimens. Proceedings of 10th ICP 2009 pp. 82-83

Gilles R. G. Monif M.D.

RECOMMENDATIONS FOR TREATMENT OF CROHN'S DISEASE

RATIONALE for RECOMENDATIONS

Crohn's disease is the concomitant functioning of three distinct, but inter-related, disease processes:

I. **Segmental immune destruction of the lining epithelium of the gastrointestinal tract and underlying submucosa (lamina propria).**

II. **Conflict between acquired and inherent immunity embedded within the submucosa and regional lymph nodes and invasive components of the microbiological flora (microbiota) of the gastrointestinal tract.**

III. Catabolic status induced by I and II

Epithelial Destruction

Epithelial destruction is the consequence of the body's immune destruction of areas of *Mycobacterium avium* subspecies *paratuberculosis* (MAP) attachment to epithelium and its subsequent antigen processing by macrophages.

This facet of Crohn's disease is the consequence of mucosal immunity having lost what is termed immune tolerance to MAP's antigenic array. To induce mucosal tolerance to its antigens, MAP infection must occur in the first few weeks of life: a time when acquired newborn immunity is close to that documented in germ-free animals.

The human gastrointestinal tract's immune system is a dynamic interplay of checks and balances. Intestinal immune regulation is achieved through opposing arms of the immune system. By their penetration, microbes initiate a pro-inflammatory T-cell response with the development of T-helper-1 (TH1, TH2 and/or TH17) cells. These pro-inflammatory cells become counterbalanced by the

- **Not all inflammatory bowel disease (IBD) is Crohn's disease. Therapy of ulcerative colitis is not the therapy of Crohn's disease. Proper diagnosis is an imperative.**

elaboration of regulatory inducible T-cells (Tregs) that have variable Foxhead Box transcription factor (Foxp3f). Treg differentiation results in production of anti-inflammatory cytokines. In experimental colitis models, suppression of TH1 and TH17 cell responses prevent the inflammatory response from developing.

If the immune system is obligated to address a replication antigen mass in the relative absence of acquired immunity, immunological memory is altered. Rather than responding to re-exposure to MAP's antigenic array by "immune tolerance" in which the cytotoxic cytokine cascade is not activated, the body's immune system responds as if this is the first time that it is so challenged.

The preponderance of MAP therapies that, directly or indirectly, can induce remissions, target effector T-cells and/ or neutralize selected cytotoxic cytokines elaborated.

MAP epithelial binding receptor sites line the entire small intestine. MAP's attachment is concentrated in areas of major fecal stasis. The immense regenerative capacity of the lining epithelium renders, quantitatively limited and widely spaced MAP antigen challenges, to be of transient significance. Increased inoculum loads and closely spaced antigen challenges eventually overwhelm the ability of the mucosa to quickly heal, resulting in a prolonged loss of the physical barrier that separated the luminal microbiota from the underlying lamina propria.

Neither viable MAP organisms nor active MAP replication are necessary for cytotoxic cytokine attack of the sites of MAP antigen attachment and its antigen processing.

Microbiological Flora of the Gastrointestinal Tract

Loss of the anatomical barrier separating bacteria, coupled with inflammation-induced reduction of the local oxygen-reduction potential, alters the microbiological hen-peck order among microbes and initiates a confrontation between invasive microbes and embedded mucosal immunity. In the absence of bacteria with enhanced virulence, epithelial reconstitution of the anatomical barrier gives leverage to mucosal immunity to terminate microbial invasion before local tissue destruction significantly advances the "anaerobic progression".

Bowel abscesses, bowel perforation and fistula are primarily the results of facultative anaerobic bacteria that have progressed within the anaerobic progression.

Inflammation introduces rigidity that the musculature of the small intestines must overcome to advance the proximal fecal contents. Some areas heal by fibrosis resulting in impaired bowel motility and ultimately stricture formation.

Metabolic Catabolism

Increased transient time, loss of mucosal surface and impaired transportation within the lamina propria deprive the body of the caloric intake and essential building blocks necessary to counterbalance the induced negative catabolic effects of Crohn's disease. The principle sites for disease induction are also prime locations for absorption of key elements necessary for acquired immunity.

RECOMMENDATIONS

Diagnosis and staging of disease are best done by a gastroenterologist.

A simple rule is that the time of a chronic disease's duration has a crude correlation with the time required for a therapeutic resolution.

PREVENTION OF EPITHELIAL DENUDEMENT and ASSOCIATED INFLAMMATION

1. The short term use of tumor necrosis factor-alpha blocking drugs or their equivalents is advocated to allow regeneration of the lining mucosa.

Prolonged use of these drugs undermines the body's immune system and creates an unnecessary risk of infection by other microbes and cancers whose limitations are governed by cell-mediated immunity.

RECOMMENDATION: Treatment with a TNF "Knockout" Drug

2. **The most important step in reconstitution of the mucosal lining is avoidance of added cytotoxic challenges**. All milk and milk-based products must be eliminated from the diet. Before the 1900s, Crohn's disease was a medical rarity. Today in the United States, between 800,000 and 1.2 million individuals have Crohn's disease or a *forme fruste* of the disease. In 2007, over 31% of bulk tank milk tested contained MAP DNA. What these figures are now is open to speculation. Viable MAP has been demonstrated in powdered milk and, in particular, in infant formula.

RECOMMENDATION: Delete from Diet of All Milk and Milk-based Products

THE SUBMUCOSA/MICROBIOTA BATTLE

Probiotics: Mucosal denudement and the resultant inflammation alter the inter-relationships between microbes within the fecal flora. To counterbalance the induced alterations in the hen-peck order among bacteria, the daily use of a probiotic is encouraged. IDI's choice of a probiotic is Lactobacillus GG.

RECOMMENDATION: Daily Administration of a Probiotic

Winning the battle for the submucosa entails limiting the number of invaders. Reclosing the epithelial barrier is a foremost consideration. Concomitant antibiotic use is often required.

An inexpensive baseline yardstick by which to judge status and need/effectiveness of antibiotic therapy is the serial use of serum C-reactive protein determinations.

The most commonly employed antibiotic combination that span the facultative anaerobic spectrum and the anaerobic spectrum of bacteria is the concomitant administration of a fluoroquinolone and metronidazole.

RECOMMENDATION: Monitored, Combined Antibacterial Antibiotic Administration

The concomitant administration of anti-mycobacterium therapy is an open issue. Such therapy is not necessary to induce temporary remission, but subsequent administration may be necessary to induce a long term remission.

Active replication of MAP is not a component necessary for active disease. MAP's fixation within the submucosa maintains the dendritic cells primed. Anti-mycobacterium drugs that target cell wall constituents may, more likely than not, be ineffective. When viable MAPs have been recovered from diseased tissues, they exist as spheroclasts (organisms without cell walls). To be effective, anti-mycobacterium therapy needs to affect either 30s or 50s ribosomes.

RECOMMENDATION: Follow up Anti-MAP Spheroclast Therapy

ENHANCEMENT OF CELL-MEDIATED IMMUNITY

Enhancement of cell-mediated immunity is one of the keys to long term remission. Individuals have achieved "cures" using just diet and self-will. In Japan, nutrition is first-line therapy.

RECOMMENDATION: Incorporate Dietary Expertise Appropriate for Attaining a Positive Anabolic Effect.

To monitor nutritional progress, the serum albumin/globulin ratio can be of assistance. If the A/G ratio is low and, particularly if the albumin component is low, dietary supplementation with specific amino acid and food sources appropriate for individuals with short bowel syndrome should be considered.

RECOMMENDATION: Aggressive Supplementation with Vitamins, Minerals, and Selected Amino Acids that Specifically Target Cell-mediated Immunity.

RECOMMENDATION: Craving for a Specific Food (if possible) should be respected.

Depression associated with loss of self-image, coupled with job related stress, adversely affects the immune system. Inducing a positive attitude in the individual to combat his or her affliction will benefit the individual's immune system. Advocate adoption of a John Wayne-like attitude and literally beat the shit out of Crohn's disease.

A useful little trick is the limited use of CoQ10. The substance can sometimes be helpful in counteracting depression of appetite that is common among individuals with Crohn's disease.

RECOMMENDATION: Initiate Steps to Diminish Stress and to Counteract Depression.

CONCLUSION

It is stated as a point of fact that "there is no current cure for Crohn's disease". In my opinion, the paralysis of critical thinking achieved by attributing Crohn's disease to "an auto-immune disease" and the reliance on pharmacological

Band-Aids to plicate human suffering have masked understanding of the elements that combine to produce disease and indirectly the potential for creative interventions.

The above are personal recommendations that should be filtered through the physician responsible for ultimate care.

Gilles R. G. Monif, M.D.